D1625875

Neuromuscular Rehabilitation in Manual and Physical Therapies

Dedicated to Tsafi, Guy, Mattan and Pinooki

Commissioning Editor: Sarena Wolfaard
Development Editor: Ailsa Laing
Project Manager: Srikumar Narayanan
Designer: Stewart Larking
Photography: Sascha Panknin
Illustration Manager: Merlyn Harvey
Illustrator: Danny Pyne

Neuromuscular Rehabilitation in Manual and Physical Therapies

Principles to Practice

Eyal Lederman DO PhD

Director, Centre for Professional Development in Manual and Physical Therapies, London, UK

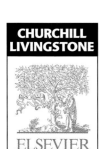

CHURCHILL LIVINGSTONE

ELSEVIER

Edinburgh   London   New York   Oxford   Philadelphia   St Louis   Sydney   Toronto   2010

CHURCHILL
LIVINGSTONE
ELSEVIER

First published 2010, © Elsevier Limited. All rights reserved.

ISBN 9780443069697
 Reprinted 2010

British Library Cataloguing in Publication Data
A catalogue record for this book is available from the British Library

Library of Congress Cataloging in Publication Data
A catalog record for this book is available from the Library of Congress

Notice
Neither the Publisher nor the Author assume any responsibility for any loss or injury and/or damage to persons or property arising out of or related to any use of the material contained in this book. It is the responsibility of the treating practitioner, relying on independent expertise and knowledge of the patient, to determine the best treatment and method of application for the patient.

The Publisher

ELSEVIER your source for books,
journals and multimedia
in the health sciences
www.elsevierhealth.com

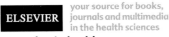

Working together to grow
libraries in developing countries

www.elsevier.com | www.bookaid.org | www.sabre.org

ELSEVIER | **BOOK AID** International | Sabre Foundation

The
Publisher's
policy is to use
**paper manufactured
from sustainable forests**

Printed in China

Contents

This book is for individuals who would like to help other individuals to recover their control of movement.

Neuromuscular rehabilitation is straightforward and uncomplicated: we all do it naturally all of the time. Throughout our lives we learn new movement patterns or recover our control after an injury. The means by which we achieve these changes are no different to neuromuscular rehabilitation. They all rely on the same neurophysiological, psychological and behavioural processes.

Neuromuscular rehabilitation integrates several branches of knowledge. They include medical, neurophysiological, psychological-behavioural and motor-control sciences as well as manual and physical therapy fields. The enormity of available information from these diverse sources can be overwhelming, in particular when trying to translate this information into a practical clinical approach. The main aim in writing this book was to collate and integrate all this information and present it in a practical, user-friendly format.

Over the years of working in clinics I have observed that neuromuscular rehabilitation of a person after joint surgery or musculoskeletal injury bears close resemblance to the clinical management of a stroke patient. It was clear to me that there is a unifying model for neuromuscular rehabilitation. However, it took a good decade and a half to put it together into a coherent and cohesive model, and one which is still being tinkered with. This unified model for neuromuscular rehabilitation is described throughout the book.

The information in the book is derived from several sources. It is a combination of my own research in the neurophysiology of manual therapy, the vast research in all the fields discussed above, my clinical experience of 23 years and my experience of teaching neuromuscular rehabilitation for the last 15 years. These experiences have made me aware of the academic and practical needs of the practitioners in this area. This is reflected in the contents of this book: it aims to bridge the gap between science and the practice of neuromuscular rehabilitation.

The contents and organization of the book

The book starts by identifying the main unifying model/principles for motor rehabilitation (Ch. 1), including the importance of a functional approach, skill- and ability-level rehabilitation and the code for neuromuscular adaptation. The following chapters discuss several areas that are relevant to neuromuscular rehabilitation. They include how movement is organized (motor control, Ch. 2) and how it is constructed from underlying control components called motor abilities (Ch. 3). These abilities are affected in various neuromuscular and musculoskeletal conditions and may, therefore, become the target of rehabilitation. Also, proprioception plays an important role in movement control and is often affected by musculoskeletal and central nervous system damage (Ch. 4).

The next important issue in rehabilitation is how to sustain the motor recovery in the long term. Chapter 5 discusses motor learning and adaptation principles and how to integrate them into the clinical management. The consequences of learning, neurophysiological/neuromuscular plasticity and adaptation are discussed in Chapter 6.

In musculoskeletal injuries the motor system reorganizes movement to prevent further damage (Ch. 7). The motor manifestation of this reorganization will be discussed as well as the indications for introducing neuromuscular rehabilitation after injury identified.

Once an individual acquires an injury, their beliefs, attitudes and behaviour may have important implications for recovery. Furthermore, the way a person uses their body or schedules their activities during the day may put them at risk for injury. These cognitive and behavioural factors are discussed in Chapter 8. This theme is continued in Chapter 9, examining non-traumatic pain conditions such as trapezius and jaw myalgia, and chronic neck pain. In this group of conditions the individual develops localized and debilitating pain without a history of tissue trauma.

Chapter 10 explores the principles of functional movement, motor control and learning/adaptation, and their use in rehabilitating patients with central nervous system damage.

Chapter 11 describes how to develop a rehabilitation programme using the key principles identified in the book. Chapter 12 describes some of the assessments and challenges of motor abilities and similarly for proprioception in Chapter 13. A summary of the book can be found in Chapter 14.

The book is supplemented by a DVD demonstrating some of the assessments and challenges of the motor abilities and their use in clinic. The movement challenges described in the book and DVD are derived from several sources. Some are research-based, others I have developed and used in clinic. Over many years of teaching I have observed professionals from different disciplines and their approach in rehabilitating movement control. Their wealth of experience and knowledge is part of this library of movement rehabilitation. It is a source book that aims to provide ideas and not recipes or treatment protocols for rehabilitation.

I hope you will find it useful.

London 2010   Prof Eyal Lederman

Introduction

This book explores how manual and physical therapists can help individuals to recover and optimize their control of movement. Musculoskeletal injury, pain experiences and central nervous system damage are all associated with diverse neuromuscular and movement control changes. The aim of this book is to provide the theoretical and practical basis for neuromuscular rehabilitation for these conditions.

This book is intended for manual and physical therapists of all disciplines (physiotherapists, osteopaths, chiropractors, sports massage therapists, etc.) who work with patients whose conditions involve the neuromuscular system. The book will also be useful for personal trainers, Alexander method teachers, Pilates instructors, postural integration teachers, Rolfing practitioners, sports trainers and individuals who experience losses in movement control.

A functional approach in rehabilitation

A functional approach in rehabilitation is the key concept underpinning the management described in this book.

Functional movement is defined here as *the unique movement repertoire of an individual*. A portion of this repertoire involves the movement behaviour associated with daily needs and demands, such as feeding, grooming, going places, etc. (*general skills*). Some movement behaviour may be partly shared with others whilst some may be unique to particular individuals; examples include physical hobbies, sports and occupational activities (*special skills*). For one person their functional repertoire may include playing tennis, for another standing on their head (yoga) or playing the piano and so on. Once a person learns a movement or a new skill it becomes a part of their movement repertoire and, therefore, their behaviour. Movement which is outside the normal repertoire of an individual will be termed here as *extra-functional* (Fig. 1.1).

Functional rehabilitation is defined here as *the process of helping a person to recover their movement capacity by using their own movement repertoire (whenever possible)*. Hence, for a person who has motor losses at the knee and is unable to walk or run, the rehabilitation will be in walking, then running, jumping and stair-climbing, etc. If this person plays tennis, this activity will also be used in the rehabilitation programme.

However, rehabilitation is likely to be less effective if the remedial movement patterns or tasks are outside the individual's experience (extra-functional). For example, it would be less helpful for a tennis player with a leg injury to be given rehabilitative exercise such as football, or leg presses in the gym or leg exercise lying on the floor (Ch. 2). For this particular patient, rehabilitation that incorporates tennis tasks is more likely to be useful. For a person who is suffering from lower back pain and enjoys yoga, a functional rehabilitation would consist of the shared functional activities (general skills), but may also include some of the upright postures from yoga (special skills). A less suitable rehabilitation approach would be to prescribe tennis to this individual. This may seem obvious; however, movement rehabilitation often prescribes extra-functional tasks such as core stability training

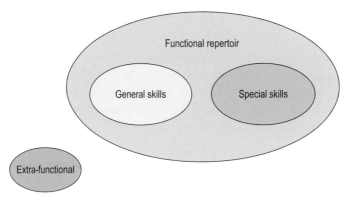

Fig. 1.1 • Functional movement represents the movement repertoire of the individual. It includes all the general activities and special skills. Extra-functional movement comprises all activities outside the individual's movement experiences.

on the floor, bracing the trunk or strength training with equipment. The question is how effective are these activities in recovering functional movement?

The introduction of extra-functional activities during rehabilitation raises some problems. Extra-functional activity or exercise requires learning a new task at a time when the patient is experiencing pain and/or loss of movement ability. This might not be the best time to enter a new exercise regime. Learning requires set-aside time, intense mental focus and physical effort. Often it means the patient has to be dependent on others for instructions and guidance during the training. A functional approach which aims to use the patient's own movement resources does not require additional learning; the cognitive demands are less taxing and do not require protracted training. Also the set-aside time for practice is more manageable for the patient. This form of rehabilitation seldom relies on any specialized exercise equipment and the remedial movement challenges are integrated into the person's daily activities. They can be practised anywhere and at any time. A functional approach is easy to apply and it empowers the patient to self-care.

There are exceptions to the functional approach in rehabilitation. There are circumstances where the patients will require specific exercises for particular motor losses; challenges which may not be provided by their functional repertoire. There are also situations where the individual is physically unable to perform functional activities. When and why the rehabilitation should stray from this model will be discussed throughout this book.

Rehabilitation levels: skill and ability level rehabilitation

Movement rehabilitation and motor normalization following injury occurs naturally for most individuals. Following injury most individuals will take physical actions that will support their spontaneous and unaided recovery. This would happen without any special knowledge or understanding of the underlying physiological principles underpinning their recovery. In this form of rehabilitation the individual is attempting to, partially or fully, execute the movement that has been lost. Attempting to walk becomes the rehabilitation for the person who lost the ability to walk. Similarly, if an individual with an arm injury is unable to reach; their repeated attempts in that pattern would often be their rehabilitation. The focus in this form of movement recovery is on the overall skill of performing the particular movement. This will be loosely referred to as *skill rehabilitation* (Ch. 9).

However, this approach does not always lead to the intended results. Individuals who are in pain or have motor losses may develop movement patterns that circumvent their losses. A patient may present with walking difficulties due to losses in the control of balance and coordination. One would imagine that by encouraging the patient to increase their walking, "walking would train balance and coordination during walking". However, what may happen is that the patient will get better at using their compensatory pattern; walking slowly, using wider gait, shorter steps, rather than truly improving their control of balance and coordination during walking.

Balance and coordination are part of several control building blocks that make up skilled movement. These building blocks are called *sensory motor abilities*. A therapeutic approach that targets the various motor abilities will be termed in this text as *re-abilitation*. At this level of rehabilitation the aim is to recover control losses associated with particular abilities. Hence, in the walking scenario described above, the rehabilitation would aim to challenge balance and coordination in dynamic and upright postures (Ch. 2).

Skill rehabilitation and re-abilitation are both clinically important and are often used in combination. However, there may be a shift of focus towards one of these particular approaches depending on the individual's condition and their phase of recovery (Ch. 9).

The code for neuromuscular adaptation

Neuromuscular rehabilitation is a straightforward process – anyone can do it. Indeed, we all do it all the time. Every day we take actions that result in movement and behaviour changes; we can self-modify our motor control. Furthermore, the neuromuscular system has the capacity for self-recovery and to reorganize in response to injury. It means that within our behaviour there are certain elements that facilitate the recovery of movement control.

In functional rehabilitation we identify five such elements that optimize neuromuscular adaptation: cognition, being active, feedback, repetition and similarity (Ch. 5). Hence, in order to learn a new task, modify our behaviour or help our system recover we need to be aware of what we are doing (cognition) and we have to actively perform the action that we aim to recover (being active). In order to correct our movement we rely on internal information from our senses or depend on guidance by someone (feedback) and we have to practise the task many times (repetition). Furthermore, the practice has to closely resemble the movement we aim to recover (similarity). Hence, to play the piano a person needs to practise the piano. However, strength training with finger weights or practising push-ups is unlikely to benefit playing the piano. The practice has to be task-specific.

The recovery of motor control can be facilitated by introducing the adaptive code element into the rehabilitation programme. It will promote a functional recovery that is more likely to benefit the patient in their daily activities. The results are more likely to be maintained in the long-term and could help to reduce the overall duration of the treatment programme.

Developing a neuromuscular rehabilitation programme

Much of the rehabilitation promoted in this book is the marrying of the three concepts discussed so far:

1. The focus on functional movement

2. The principle of skill/ability level rehabilitation

3. The code for motor adaptation (Ch. 9).

Through a simple three-step process the therapist decides which level of rehabilitation will be used and applies the motor adaptation elements to the treatment programme. Many of the remedial challenges are selected from the patient's own movement repertoire. It really is that simple.

The beauty of it all is that these principles can be applied to any condition in which the neuromuscular system is implicated:

Conditions with an intact motor system

- Neuromuscular changes associated with musculoskeletal injuries, sports injuries, post surgery, back pain and other musculoskeletal pain conditions (Ch. 7)
- Conditions where certain behaviours impede recovery or may lead to injury or pain (Ch. 8)
- Non-traumatic pain conditions, such as trapezius myalgia, chronic neck pain and painful jaw (Ch. 9).

Conditions where there is damage to the central nervous system

- Stroke, head trauma and post central nervous system (CNS) surgery and all the degenerative conditions (Ch. 10).

The main difference in managing these conditions is in the magnitude of losses, the duration of recovery and the extent of potential recovery.

Summary points

- Neuromuscular rehabilitation aims to help the individual recover their movement control.
- Functional movement is the movement repertoire of an individual.
- Functional movement is individual-specific.

- Functional rehabilitation uses the patient's own movement repertoire to help him/her to recover their movement losses.
- The rehabilitation promoted in this book has three basic recurring concepts:

  1. It aims to be functional.
  2. It uses the skill/ability level rehabilitation concept.
  3. It uses the learning/adaptation code to optimize motor control changes.

Motor control

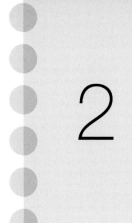

The motor system organizes and controls skeletal muscle activation during movement, posture and the musculoskeletal aspect of behaviour and expression. The motor system spans the whole of the central nervous system (CNS). It is not a discrete functional or anatomical entity.

This chapter will examine how movement is organized and the implications it has for neuromuscular rehabilitation.

The organization for movement

Imagine an action such as reaching for a cup. For that action we need to collect information from all our senses about our body and the environment.[1–3] We can than select the most suitable response to get hold of the cup. Once a decision has been made a motor command ensues,[2] muscles are activated and a reaching movement is the outcome. Some elements of the motor process will be at conscious level, "that we are reaching for the cup", while a larger proportion will remain at a subconscious level,[4] such as the fine postural adjustments that precede the action. Hence, any movement has conscious and reflexive elements and identifiable stages (Fig. 2.1):

- Integration stage
- Motor stage
- Sensory stage.

These stages should be viewed as a process with multiple sub-events rather than separate entities.[5]

The integration stage

Once an individual has decided to take an action the role of the integration stage is to prepare the neuromuscular system for the execution of the associated movement. Within the integration stage there are two processes that have important implications for neuromuscular rehabilitation. The first is how movement is encoded by the motor centres for future use and the second is how movement errors are identified.

Motor programmes and movement parameters

Our movement repertoire is stored within the central nervous system as motor programmes. They are not centre-specific and seem to be stored throughout the central nervous system, including the spinal cord.[6–10]

The motor programmes are believed to be generalized schemes containing information about the *movement sequences* and their goals rather than specific muscle sequences.[2] Writing is an example of such a generalized scheme. A word can be written in many different ways; it can be written fast or slow, from different angles, in larger or small amplitudes, whilst sitting or standing, or even in completely new, unrehearsed situations. It can be written with the non-dominant hand, with each foot and even with the pen held between the teeth. A mild stroke patient once demonstrated to me how she could write beautiful calligraphy with the affected arm/side. She would hold the pen in the

Fig. 2.1 • The motor system as a process. The inner circle represents processes occurring at reflexive, sub-awareness level.

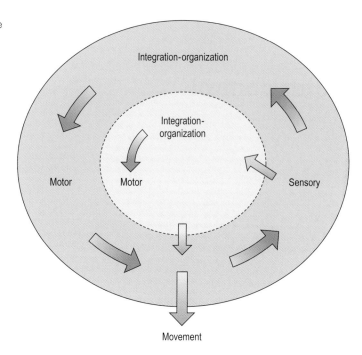

hand; stiffen her arm and write by moving her whole body. In these writing examples, the schema for writing is executable by any part of the body because it is not specific to any particular muscle group.[11–15]

Once a task has been learned the movement sequences become more robust to change, e.g. a person's handwriting is unique and will remain largely unchanged through life. However, certain factors such as the force, speed, range/size of the writing can be changed at any time.[2] By modifying these movement parameters any task can be performed with infinite variations.[11–15]

The movement parameters have an important role in neuromuscular rehabilitation. It has been demonstrated that in musculoskeletal injury or in pain conditions the motor system "narrows" these movement parameters. This reorganization of movement control is a protection strategy which serves to alleviate some of the stresses imposed on the damaged tissues (Ch. 7). For example, a person suffering from lower back pain may demonstrate trunk muscle force losses,[21–23] reduced movement speed,[23–26] reduced endurance,[16–20] changes in the normal timing and duration of synergists in the trunk muscles,[27–37] changes in coordinated movement of the pelvis and thorax,[24,25] reduced postural stability[31,34,38–40] and loss of the ability to respond to sudden postural changes.[28–36,41] Hence, a person with back pain will often display a posture and gait which is different from their usual patterns. The normal schemes for walking are still preserved, but the movement parameters have changed. This motor reorganization will also influence certain building-blocks of movement called *motor abilities* (see Ch. 3).

The comparator system

Imagine that while lifting the cup it slipped from your hand resulting in immediate reflexive grasp. The error detection is carried out by the comparator system.

Once a movement pattern has been selected the efferent commands are transmitted to the spinal motor centres to initiate muscle activity. At the same time a copy of this information (*efferent or efference copy*) is transmitted internally to be processed by the comparator system (Fig. 2.2). Here, the information from the efference copy and the information from the sensory inputs are matched against the expected outcome of the action.[2,42–45] Any mismatch will result in motor reorganization and correction of the movement.

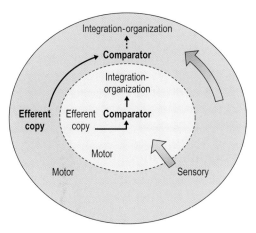

Fig. 2.2 • The comparator system identifies movement irregularities/errors.

The comparator system reduces the processing demands placed on the CNS by selectively drawing attention to movement, but only when there is a change from the norm. As long as the information is similar it will remain at a low priority within the overall motor processes. Hence, many of our familiar daily activities (e.g. walking) remain below consciousness until we make a mistake (e.g. tripping).

When learning a new task it will be acquired through a process of making errors and their correction. This error detection is carried out by the comparator system. This detection process is only functional during "active" rather than passive movement. It implies that motor learning will be more effective in rehabilitation approaches where the person is active and concurrently correcting their movement, in comparison to passive approaches.

The comparator system also plays a role in proprioception. When we move our limbs there is a sense of their weight and the effort that is required to move them. This sense of effort is believed to be derived internally by central processes (comparator) and not from the proprioceptors.[2,43,45–47] It has been hypothesized that during motor development we learn to associate the effort with movement sensations (proprioception). Eventually, the sense of effort becomes a proprioceptive signal in its own right.[48]

The sense of effort, as a source of feedback, is only present during active rather than passive movement. Hence, during active movement proprioceptive acuity increases, compared to the same movement being performed passively. It implies that more effective proprioceptive rehabilitation can be achieved by active rather than passive movement approaches. The full clinical implication of this phenomenon is further discussed in Chapters 4 and 13.

The motor stage

The motor stage is the culmination of the selection of movement schemes and the transmission of these efferent commands to the spinal motor centres.

One way to visualize the motor output is to imagine a person wearing an electromyographic (EMG) body-suit. This suit would have numerous EMG electrodes that could record the motor activity from every single muscle or, even better, from every motor unit in the body. Furthermore, imagine that the suit is covered by minute lights that would represent the intensity of the underlying motor events. Areas with high motor activity will be represented by brighter light and vice-versa. If this was possible, we would probably see a psychedelic light show throughout the body, with different areas lighting at different intensities – the motor output is a whole body event. These patterns would change on a moment-to-moment basis as the person moves or even while they are still.[49]

The EMG suit would probably demonstrate that movement is achieved by shifting tension gradients throughout the body (Fig. 2.3). In order to move

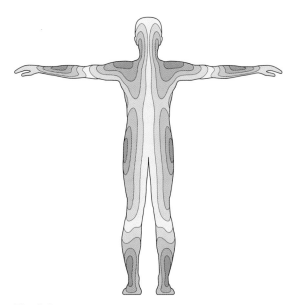

Fig. 2.3 • Dynamic tensional fields produce movement. These fields change continuously on a moment-to-moment basis and are unlikely to repeat themselves.

the arm to the mouth, tension develops in the anterior aspect of the upper limb, while on the opposite side the tension in the limb diminishes. The way to imagine it is as broad and dynamic *tensional fields*, rather than separate and individual muscles. These fields are widespread and are continuously varying in their intensities. Interestingly, most of the proprioceptors in our body are tension receptors (except for the skin, which has pressure receptors). It seems that during movement the nervous system "sees" areas of varying tensions rather than individual tendons, joint capsules or muscles.

> ## Clinical note
>
> The concept of tensional field can help us to make an important clinical shortcut: there is no need to know the complex and exact anatomy of muscles for effective neuromuscular rehabilitation. The focus is on movement capacity and not on individual muscles.

The complexity of recruitment

The recruitment of muscle is composed of highly complex patterns. Imagine a simple movement such as turning the head. Some muscles will be recruited to produce the tensional field necessary to rotate the head; meanwhile all the antagonistic muscles will reduce their tensional field. Concurrently, muscles bilaterally will increase in co-tension to prevent the head from falling sideways (Fig. 2.4a). These muscles have to dynamically stabilize the movement while sharing some element in the execution of the turning motion. As the head moves beyond the centre of its gravity the action of these muscles will reverse. The antagonists develop low-level eccentric tension to counter the weight of the head; the original movers will drop in tension and so on. If we were to describe every muscle activity in this simple movement it would probably fill the whole of this book and beyond. This complexity is depicted in Figure 2.4b.

It has been demonstrated that every task or movement we perform will never exactly repeat itself.[50–55] Throughout life "every breath you take, every step you make" and every heart beat is different. Yet, in all this complexity we somehow produce movement that is definable, precise and is unique to ourselves. It is now suggested that such

variability is an essential healthy aspect of biological systems and that during injury and disease processes this variability tends to be diminished.[50,53] Such loss of variability was demonstrated during walking in patients with chronic lower back pain. When the trunk was perturbed they seemed to have a narrower selection of postural responses to any sudden movement.[24,25]

Goal-orientated movement

Movement is organized with an overall goal or purpose: we reach for a cup, hit a ball or walk to a location; but we don't set out to move our limbs, move a joint or contract a muscle.[56]

For an outsider watching a person performing a task it can be broken down into the action or movement and its outcome, the goal.[57] Once we learn how to achieve a certain goal, the action and the outcome are integrated to become a unified automatic response. They are represented internally as images of the goal[57,58] When we perform an action or task, thinking of the outcome/goal triggers the execution of the associated movement.[59] Interestingly, 7-month-old infants favour learning by imitating movements that have obvious goals but not those that have ambiguous goals.[60,61]

The whole body is organized to take part in the goal of the movement including all the anticipatory postural adjustments that precede it.[62] Different parts of the body tend to "lead the way" during goal movement. The arms for reaching or throwing, the

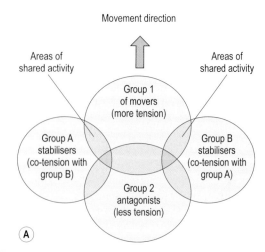

Fig. 2.4 • A, "Simplified complexity" in tensional fields. Shaded circles represent tension created by muscle groups.

(Continued)

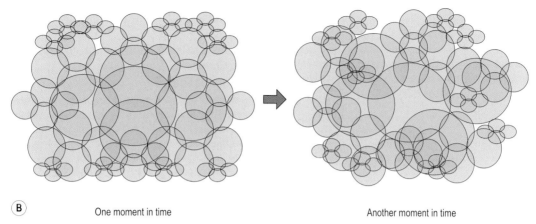

(B)
One moment in time   Another moment in time

Fig. 2.4—cont'd. B, Complexity is movement.

legs for kicking or stepping over an obstacle and the head leads in the initiation of walking and turning. Head movement is also led by our senses;[63] turning the head to a sudden noise, looking up or bending forward to smell or taste. The odd one out is the trunk: it rarely leads in movement. In rehabilitation of back conditions should the trunk/spine be a focus of movement training or should it be engaged within the overall movement goal?

Clinical note

Movement control should be associated with its goals during rehabilitation, i.e. rehabilitation should use goal-orientated and task-specific movements. Movement where the body itself is the goal may be less effective in recovering motor control (see also Internal and external focus and learning, Ch. 5).

Task-dependent muscle recruitment

The muscle recruitment will vary considerably from one task to another.[64–69] For example, the trunk muscles will display completely different activation patterns during standing, walking, reaching to the sides or forward, bending or lifting or any other imaginable movement.[70,71] Furthermore, even within the same task, changes in the underlying movement parameters and other factors will influence the complex recruitment of muscles. They include:

- *The force* – movement which is similar but at a varying force will change the muscle recruitment.[35]

- *The amplitude of movement* – how far a person reaches changes the pattern of trunk muscle activation.[35,36]

- *The rate/speed of movement* – changing the speed of movement will also change recruitment patterns.[72] For example, there is different trunk muscles recruitment during slow or fast arm movement.[30]

- *The position or direction* – slight variations in underlying posture/position during movement will change overall patterns of muscle recruitment. For example, different positions during exercise will recruit different patterns in the trunk muscles.[68] Likewise, movement of the body in a different direction will change the pattern of activation of the abdominal muscles.[36,73,74]

- *Contact/contact-free movement (open-closed kinetic chains)* – muscle recruitment is different if movement is contact-free (e.g. waving your arm) from movement where the body makes contact with another base, such as the floor, wall or an object.[75–77] Hence, muscle recruitment in the arms is different during push-ups (contact) than the same arms movement performed standing in space without contact. Interestingly, most of our body is involved in a mixture of these two contact patterns, except for the head, which is invariably contact-free. Does this mean that functional rehabilitation of the neck should focus on contact-free head movements?

- *Pain* – the experience, anticipation or fear of pain will influence the muscle recruitment patterns.[21,24,25,31,78–81]

The movement should be practised in different positions, forces and speeds, and using both contact and non-contact patterns. This would aim to account for the infinite variability that exists in normal daily movement. Rehabilitation should not be restricted to set movement patterns with minimal variability or focused on particular muscles (e.g. weight-training or performing biceps curls). Such an approach will result in the patient's learning to control muscles in relation to these specific tasks, in patterns which are unlikely to carry over to other tasks (see Similarity principle and transfer, Ch. 5).

The sensory stage

During movement the motor system collects information about internal physical events as well as information from the environment.[3,44,83] This is provided by two feedback systems:

- Proprioceptors – which provide information about internal mechanical events
- Exteroceptors (vision and vestibular/hearing) – which provide information about the environment.

When we reach for an object our movement is organized in response to the information provided by these two feedback systems. Information from vision is used to estimate the distance and the size of the object to be handled.[2] The proprioceptive and visual information is integrated with vestibular information to maintain the body balanced and upright during the reaching task.[84-86] The skin receptors signal the contact of the fingers with the object and provide information about its mass, size and texture. Further information arrives from receptors in the muscles and joints, indicating the position of the arm in space and the relationship of different body masses to each other; the speed and direction of movement and the force of contraction (sense of effort).[47,48,87-94]

The processing of sensory information occurs both at a conscious and subconscious levels.[94-98] However, much of this extensive information is processed at a subconscious/reflexive level, unless we draw our attention to any element of it.

Role of proprioception

Proprioception has several important roles in motor processes. It provides:

- feedback for immediate adjustments and refinement of movement

- feedback for motor learning
- replenishment of pre-existing motor programmes.

Motor control relies on proprioception for the final adjustment, refinement and synchronization of complex movement.[99,100] It also provides information if the movement strays away from what is intended, e.g. walking and tripping. Proprioception losses may lead to unrefined and inaccurate movement, and are believed to predispose the individual to recurrent injury (see Discussion, Ch. 4).

During very rapid movements the processing of sensory feedback is too slow to allow correction of the ongoing movement.[42,46,101–106] This is seen in activities such as walking, jumping, running, fast ballistic movements, typing or playing a musical instrument. In these movements the pre-programmed motor patterns precede the sensory feedback.[102] The motor system, therefore, has to rely on the information gathered before the onset of, rather than from the instantaneous feedback during, the movement. Consequently, the correction of the movement occurs close to or at the termination of movement. For example, during running and jumping, the activation of leg extensors precedes the foot contact with the ground by about 150–180 m. This fact has implications for preventing injuries in sports. Since the afferent transmission time within the CNS is fairly fixed, improving proprioception is unlikely to reduce injuries that occur during high-velocity movements. However, injuries may be prevented by changing the way the person performs the movement (see Discussions on task-behaviour and correctness of movement, Chs 7 & 8).

Our mind is "shaped" by our experiences and our experiences are formed by our senses. Proprioception, therefore, is essential for learning or recovering control of movement.[46] Therefore, partial or complete losses of proprioception may slow down rehabilitation. Indeed, re-abilitation of stroke patients with sensory loss may be more difficult than of those with an intact sensory system.[107,108]

The importance of proprioception for motor learning can be also seen in medical conditions in which a subject loses all their proprioception (often due to damage to the dorsal column of the spinal cord).[109] Under these circumstances, the individual is still capable of performing tasks learned before the onset of their condition.[110] However, they may find it difficult to modify the task or learn a new one. In one such documented case, the subject could still drive the car he used before his illness, but could not drive a new car as he was unable to learn the fine adjustments needed for the new mechanical situation.[111]

The refinement of the pre-stored programmes is also dependent on proprioception, without which the motor programmes deteriorate over time.[112] This is experienced in everyday circumstances when attempting to carry out a physical activity that has not been rehearsed for a long time (e.g. cycling). A few "goes" are usually needed to refine the stored programme.

Proprioception also plays an important role in body-image and the sense of self. These topics are relevant to behaviour and movement control, but are outside the scope of this book (for full discussion see: Lederman 2005 *The Science and Practice of Manual Therapy*, Section 3).

Proprioceptors

Proprioceptors (mechanoreceptors) are found in the skin, muscles, tendons, ligaments and joints (see Table 2.1 for groups of mechanoreceptors and their actions).

Afferent fibres from mechanoreceptors converge segmentally on the dorsal horn of the spinal cord. This anatomical segmental relationship is lost within the spinal cord. The afferent fibres tend to diverge in an ascending and descending manner, over several segments, synapsing with different neuronal pools and spinal interneurons. This sharing of afferents by motor centres has also been demonstrated in the cortex.[132] Hence, many synergistic muscle groups share common afferent inputs.[133–135] This means that spindle afferents from one group of muscles supply the motorneurons of the muscle in which they are embedded, as well as other synergistic muscles.[136]

The functional implications of the diverging synaptic connections can be demonstrated by tapping the biceps tendon. When tapped, the reflex response spreads to muscles as far away as the pectoralis major, triceps, deltoid and hypothenar muscles.[137] Similarly, tapping the tendon of lateral oblique brings about a reflex muscle response in all the abdominal muscles.[138] Even passive movement of the shoulder influences the gain of the motoneurons supplying muscles of the hand.[132] This physical organization has functional logic. Performance of a task involves total body movement occurring over many joints and muscle groups. The information about activity

Table 2.1 Mechanoreceptor groups, their anatomical location and function.[3,62,86, 113–131]

	Receptor	Location	Function	Interesting stuff
Muscle tendon unit	Spindle afferents Ia & II	Muscle II afferents are situated at both sides of the Ia afferent (on average, there is only one secondary to one primary as some spindles contain only primary afferents)	Feedback about length, velocity, acceleration, deceleration and minimally about the force of contraction	The more refined the function of the muscle, the greater the number of spindles per unit weight of the muscle. The detection of force is delegated to the Golgi tendon organ
	Golgi tendon organ	Tendons close to the musculotendinous junction	Feedback about dynamic changes in the force of contraction. They are not stretch receptors, as is sometimes believed. Contraction of a single muscle fibre to which they are attached will bring about an increase in their discharge	In some muscles, the capsule of the spindle is fused or continues to form the capsule of the Golgi tendon organ. They are connected to 10–20 muscle fibres and are generally not affected by mechanical events in other muscle fibres
	Groups III & IV	Muscle	Chemosensitive. Information about metabolic changes and muscle damage/ inflammation	Have an indirect influence on proprioception, via spinal and higher centres. Can influence the sensitivity of the spindle afferents
Joints	Groups I & II	Joint capsules and ligaments	Range, speed and position of the joint. Group I (dynamic and static, low threshold, slow adapting), Group II (dynamic, fast adapting)	Most joint afferents are only responsive to a movement arc of about 15–20°
	Group III	Joint capsules and ligaments	Information about dynamic events in joints. High threshold receptors that become sensitized by extreme joint position or joint injury/ inflammation	A lowering of threshold (sensitization) takes place at the receptor peripherally, but also centrally within the spinal cord
	Group IV	Joint capsules and ligaments	Nociceptors. Convey information about excessive stresses at the joint. Become sensitized in joint inflammation	Although they are not true mechanoreceptors, movements activates some group VI, albeit providing a poor sense of joint position. Receptor sensitization by peripheral and central processes

Table 2.1 Mechanoreceptor groups, their anatomical location and function—Cont'd

	Receptor	Location	Function	Interesting stuff
Skin mechano receptors	Five types skin receptors: two fast-adapting and three slow-adapting receptors	Skin	Convey information about the contact and surface texture of objects. Contribute to fast reflexive gripping when an object is slipping through the hand. Skin tension contributes to joint movement sense. More sensitive to dynamic rather than static mechanical stimulation	When skin mechanoreceptors near the nail bed are stimulated it elicits a sensation of flexion at the distal interphalangeal joint. Interestingly, the perioral area of the human face lacks any proprioceptors except for skin mechanoreceptors which play a role in the position of the lips

in one group of muscles has to be conveyed centrally to be integrated with all the other spinal motoneurons and higher centres taking part in the movement.

>
> ## Clinical note
>
> The divergence of afferents has important implications for proprioceptive rehabilitation. It suggests that localized, joint/muscle-specific rehabilitation may not be as effective in recovering control losses as rehabilitation of whole movement patterns.

Nociception as feedback

When we are in pain we move differently. Nociception is an important feedback system from the body to inform us about tissue damage or the potential for it. In response to the experience of pain the motor system will reorganize movement that is less physically stressful.

Psychological and behavioural factors related to the pain experience will have profound effects on movement control. In many musculoskeletal conditions the intensity of the pain experience and/or the resultant fear of it will often reflect in more extensive motor reorganization (Ch. 8).[23,31,38,]

> ## Clinical note
>
> Injured individuals and those in pain will select movement patterns that are beneficial for them. It raises the question, when does this positive protection strategy become a dysfunction, and at what point should there be a therapeutic intervention to change it? These issues will be discussed more fully in Chapter 7.

Summary points

- The motor system organizes and controls skeletal muscle activation during movement, posture and the musculoskeletal aspect of behaviour and expression.
- Motor processes have identifiable phases: integration, motor and feedback stages.
- Movement is stored as a scheme rather than as a fixed representation of the movement or specific muscle sequences.
- All movement is goal or task orientated and this should be reflected during rehabilitation.
- Rehabilitate whole movement – focusing on single muscles or muscle chains is not effective or essential for recovering motor control.

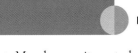
- Muscle recruitment changes according to the ongoing task or changes in the movement parameters.
- The motor system integrates proprioception and exteroception for the organization of movement.
- Proprioception provides information about internal mechanical events in the body.
- Proprioception is used by the motor system for the refinement of movement, motor learning and replenishing existing programmes.
- Pain is also feedback that has a profound influence on movement control.
- The aim of this chapter was to demonstrate the complexity of the motor output.
- This complexity promotes a functional approach in rehabilitation where the focus is on whole, goal-orientated movement.
- "Integrate in order to coordinate".

References

[1] Henry FM, Rogers DE. Increased response latency for complicated movements in a 'memory drum' theory of neuromotor reaction. Res Q 1960;31:448–458.

[2] Schmidt RA, Lee TD. Motor control and learning. 4th ed UK: Human Kinetics; 2005.

[3] Williams HG. Neurological concepts and perceptual-motor behavior. In: Brown RC, Cratty BJ, editors. New perspective of man in action. Englewood Cliffs, NJ: Prentice Hall; 1969.

[4] Soon CS, Brass M, Heinze HJ, et al. Unconscious determinants of free decisions in the human brain. Nat Neurosci 2008;11 (5):543–545. [Epub 2008 Apr 13].

[5] Hermsdörfer J, Hagl E, Nowak DA. Deficits of anticipatory grip force control after damage to peripheral and central sensorimotor systems. Hum Mov Sci 2004;23(5):643–662.

[6] Adkins DL, Boychuk J, Remple MS, et al. Motor training induces experience-specific patterns of plasticity across motor cortex and spinal cord. J Appl Physiol 2006;101:1776–1782.

[7] Barrière G, Leblond H, Provencher J, et al. Prominent role of the spinal central pattern generator in the recovery of locomotion after partial spinal cord injuries. J Neurosci 2008; 28(15):3976–3987.

[8] Fouad K, Tse A. Adaptive changes in the injured spinal cord and their role in promoting functional recovery. Neurol Res 2008; 30(1):17–27.

[9] Grillner S, Zanggar P. How detailed is the central pattern generator for locomotion? Brain Res 1975;88:367–371.

[10] Zehr EP. Training-induced adaptive plasticity in human somatosensory reflex path. J Appl Physiol 2006;101:1783–1794.

[11] Buchanan JJ, Zihlman K, Ryu YU, et al. Learning and transfer of a relative phase pattern and a joint amplitude ratio in a rhythmic multijoint. J Mot Behav 2007; 39(1):49–67.

[12] Dean NJ, Kovacs AJ, Shea CH. Transfer of movement sequences: bigger is better. Acta Psychol (Amst) 2008;127(2):355–368.

[13] LaFiandra M, Wagenaar RC, Holt KG, et al. How do load carriage and walking speed influence trunk coordination and stride parameters? J Biomech 2003;36(1):87–95.

[14] Meuhlbauer T, Panzer S, Shea CH. The transfer of movement sequences: effects of decreased and increased load. Q J Exp Psychol (Colchester) 2007;60(6):770–778.

[15] Wilde H, Shea CH. Proportional and nonproportional transfer of movement sequences. Q J Exp Psychol (Colchester) 2006; 59(9):1626–1647.

[16] Airaksinen O, Herno A, Kaukanen E, et al. Density of lumbar muscles 4 years after decompressive spinal surgery. Eur Spine J 1996;5(3):193–197.

[17] Hides JA, Stokes MJ, Saide M, et al. Evidence of lumbar multifidus muscle wasting ipsilateral to symptoms in patients with acute/subacute low back pain. Spine 1994;19(2): 165–172.

[18] Hides JA, Richardson CA, Jull GA. Multifidus muscle recovery is not automatic after resolution of acute, first-episode low back pain. Spine 1996; 21(23):2763–2769.

[19] Ng JK, Richardson CA, Kippers V, et al. Relationship between muscle fiber composition and functional capacity of back muscles in healthy subjects and patients with back pain. J Orthop Sports Phys Ther 1998; 27(6):389–402.

[20] Shirado O, Ito T, Kaneda K, Strax TE. Flexion-relaxation phenomenon in the back muscles. A comparative study between healthy subjects and patients with chronic low back pain. Am J Phys Med Rehabil 1995;74(2): 139–144.

[21] Lamoth CJ, Stins JF, Pont M, et al. Effects of attention on the control of locomotion in individuals with chronic low back pain. J Neuroeng Rehabil 2008;5:13.

[22] Shirado O, Ito T, Kaneda K, Strax TE. Concentric and eccentric strength of trunk muscles: influence of test postures on strength and characteristics of patients with chronic low-back pain. Arch Phys Med Rehabil 1995;76 (7):604–611.

[23] Thomas JS, France CR, Lavender SA, et al. Effects of fear of movement on spine velocity and acceleration after recovery

from low back pain. Spine 2008;33(5):564–570.

[24] Lamoth CJ, Daffertshofer A, Meijer OG, et al. How do persons with chronic low back pain speed up and slow down? Trunk-pelvis coordination and lumbar erector spinae activity during gait. Gait Posture 2006;23(2):230–239.

[25] Lamoth CJ, Meijer OG, Daffertshofer A, et al. Effects of chronic low back pain on trunk coordination and back muscle activity during walking: changes in motor control. Eur Spine J 2006; 15(1):23–40.

[26] Zedka M, Prochazka A, Knight B, et al. Voluntary and reflex control of human back muscles during induced pain. J Physiol 1999;520 (Pt 2):591–604.

[27] Cholewicki J, Panjabi MM, Khachatryan A. Stabilizing function of trunk flexor-extensor muscles around a neutral spine posture. Spine 1997;22(19): 2207–2212.

[28] Hodges PW, Richardson CA. Inefficient muscular stabilization of the lumbar spine associated with low back pain. A motor control evaluation of transversus abdominis. Spine 1996;21(22): 2640–2650.

[29] Hodges PW, Richardson CA. Delayed postural contraction of transversus abdominis in low back pain associated with movement of the lower limb. Spinal Disord 1998;11(1):46–56.

[30] Hodges PW, Richardson CA. Altered trunk muscle recruitment in people with low back pain with upper limb movement at different speeds. Arch Phys Med Rehabil 1999;80(9):1005–1012.

[31] Hodges PW, Moseley GL, Gabrielsson A, Gandevia SC. Experimental muscle pain changes feedforward postural responses of the trunk muscles. Exp Brain Res 2003;151(2): 262–271.

[32] MacDonald DA, Moseley GL, Hodges PW. The lumbar multifidus: Does the evidence support clinical beliefs? Man Ther 2006;11(4):254–263. [Epub 2006 May 23].

[33] O'Sullivan P, Twomey L, Allison G, et al. Altered patterns of abdominal muscle activation in patients with chronic low back pain. Aust J Physiother 1997; 43(2):91–98.

[34] Radebold A, Cholewicki J, Polzhofer GK, Greene HS. Impaired postural control of the lumbar spine is associated with delayed muscle response times in patients with chronic idiopathic low back pain. Spine 2001;26(7): 724–730.

[35] Thomas JS, France CR, Sha D, Vander Wiele N, Moenter S, Swank K. The effect of chronic low back pain on trunk muscle activations in target reaching movements with various loads. Spine 2007;32(26):E801–E808.

[36] Thomas JS, France CR. Pain-related fear is associated with avoidance of spinal motion during recovery from low back pain. Spine 2007;32(16):E460–E466.

[37] Van Dieen JH, Cholewicki J, Radebold A. Trunk muscle recruitment patterns in patients with low back pain enhance the stability of the lumbar spine. Spine 2003;28(8):834–841.

[38] Bouche K, Stevens V, Cambier D, et al. Comparison of postural control in unilateral stance between healthy controls and lumbar discectomy patients with and without pain. Eur Spine J 2006;15(4):423–432.

[39] della Volpe R, Popa T, Ginanneschi F, et al. Changes in coordination of postural control during dynamic stance in chronic low back pain patients. Gait Posture 2006;24(3):349–355.

[40] Mok NW, Brauer SG, Hodges PW. Hip strategy for balance control in quiet standing is reduced in people with low back pain. Spine 2004;29(6): E107–E112.

[41] Luoto S, Taimela S, Hurri H, et al. Psychomotor speed and postural control in chronic low back pain patients. A controlled follow-up study. Spine 1996; 21(22):2621–2627.

[42] Laszlo JI, Bairstow PJ. Accuracy of movement, peripheral feedback and efferent copy. J Mot Behav 1971;3:241–252.

[43] McCloskey DI, Gandevia SC. Role of inputs from skin, joints and muscles and of corollary discharges, in human discriminatory tasks. In: Gordon G, editor. Active touch. Oxford: Pergamon Press; 1978. p. 177–188.

[44] Smith JL. Kinesthesis: a model for movement feedback. In: Brown RC, Cratty BJ, editors. New perspective of man in action. Englewood Cliffs, NJ: Prentice Hall; 1969.

[45] Von-Holst E. Relations between the central nervous system and the peripheral organs. Br J Anim Behav 1954;2:89–94.

[46] Laszlo JI. Training of fast tapping with reduction of kinaesthetic, tactile, visual and auditory sensations. Q J Exp Psychol 1967;19:344–349.

[47] Gandevia SC, Smith JL, Crawford M, et al. Motor commands contribute to human position sense. J Physiol 2006;571 (Pt 3):703–710.

[48] Walsh LD, Allen TJ, Gandevia SC, Proske U. Effect of eccentric exercise on position sense at the human forearm in different postures. J Appl Physiol 2006;100(4): 1109–1116.

[49] Patla AE, Ishac MG, Winter DA. Anticipatory control of center of mass and joint stability during voluntary arm movement from a standing posture: interplay between active and passive control. Exp Brain Res 2002; 143(3):318–327.

[50] Bartlett R, Wheat J, Robins M. Is movement variability important for sports biomechanists? Sports Biomech 2007;6(2):224–243.

[51] Haggard P, Hutchinson K, Stein J. Patterns of coordinated multi-joint movement. Exp Brain Res 1995;107(2):254–266.

[52] Hausdorff JM, Peng CK, Ladin Z, et al. Is walking a random walk? Evidence for long-range correlations in stride interval of human gait. J Appl Physiol 1995;78(1):349–358.

[53] Stergiou N, Harbourne R, Cavanaugh J. Optimal movement variability: a new theoretical perspective for

neurologic physical therapy. J Neurol Phys Ther 2006; 30(3):120–129.

[54] van Beers RJ, Baraduc P, Wolpert DM. Role of uncertainty in sensorimotor control. Philos Trans R Soc Lond B Biol Sci 2002;357(1424):1137–1145.

[55] Yamamoto Y, Hughson RL. On the fractal nature of heart rate variability in humans: effects of data length and beta-adrenergic blockade. Am J Physiol 1994; 266(1 Pt 2):R40–R49.

[56] Hughlings Jackson J. On the comparative study of disease of the nervous system. Brit Med J 1889;17:355–362.

[57] Elsner B, Hommel B. Effect anticipation and action control. J Exp Psychol Hum Percept Perform 2001;27(1):229–240.

[58] Hommel B. The cognitive representation of action: automatic integration of perceived action effects. Psychol Res 1996;59(3):176–186.

[59] Koch I, Keller R, Prinz W. The ideomotor approach to action control: implication for skilled performance. Int J Sport Exerc Psychol 2004;2:362–375.

[60] Elsner B. Infants' imitation of goal-directed actions: the role of movements and action effects. Acta Psychol (Amst) 2007; 124(1):44–59.

[61] Hamlin JK, Hallinan EV, Woodward AL. Do as I do: 7-month-old infants selectively reproduce others' goals. Dev Sci 2008;11(4):487–494.

[62] Rosenbaum DA, Meulenbroek RGJ, Vaughan J. What is the point of motor planning? Int J Sport Exerc Psychol 2004;2:439–469.

[63] Corneil BD, Munoz DP, Olivier E. Priming of head premotor circuits during oculomotor preparation. J Neurophysiol 2007; 97(1):701–714.

[64] Carpenter RSH. Neurophysiology. London: Edward Arnold; 1990.

[65] Decker MJ, Tokish JM, Ellis HB, et al. Subscapularis muscle activity during selected rehabilitation exercises. Am J Sports Med 2003;31(1):126–134.

[66] Doemges F, Rack PMH. Changes in the stretch reflex of the human first interosseous muscle during different tasks. J Physiol 1992;447:563–573.

[67] Hore J, McCloskey DI, Taylor JL. Task-dependent changes in gain of the reflex response to imperceptible perturbations of joint position in man. J Physiol 1990;429:309–321.

[68] McGill SM, Grenier S, Kavcic N, et al. Coordination of muscle activity to assure stability of the lumbar spine. J Electromyogr Kinesiol 2003;13(4):353–359.

[69] Weiss EJ, Flanders M. Muscular and postural synergies of the human hand. J Neurophysiol 2004;92(1):523–535.

[70] Andersson EA, Oddsson LI, Grundstrom H, et al. EMG activities of the quadratus lumborum and erector spinae muscles during flexion-relaxation and other motor tasks. Clin Biomech (Bristol, Avon) 1996;11:392–400.

[71] Kavcic N, Grenier S, McGill SM. Determining the stabilizing role of individual torso muscles during rehabilitation exercises. Spine 2004;29(11):1254–1265.

[72] Chumanov ES, Heiderscheit BC, Thelen DG. The effect of speed and influence of individual muscles on hamstring mechanics during the swing phase of sprinting. J Biomech 2007; 40(16):3555–3562.

[73] Carpenter MG, Tokuno CD, Thorstensson A, et al. Differential control of abdominal muscles during multi-directional support-surface translations in man. Exp Brain Res 2008;188(3):445–455. [Epub Apr 29].

[74] Urquhart DM, Hodges PW, Story IH. Postural activity of the abdominal muscles varies between regions of these muscles and between body positions. Gait Posture 2005;22(4): 295–301.

[75] Stensdotter AK, Dalén T, Holmgren C. Knee angle and force vector-dependent variations in open and closed kinetic chain for M. popliteus activation. J Orth Stensdotter Op Res 2008;26(2):217–224.

[76] Stensdotter AK, Hodges PW, Mellor R, et al. Quadriceps activation in closed and in open kinetic chain exercise. Med Sci Sports Exerc 2003;35(12): 2043–2047.

[77] Wilk KE, Escamilla RF, Fleisig GS, Barrentine SW, Andrews JR, Boyd ML. A comparison of tibiofemoral joint forces and electromyographic activity during open and closed kinetic chain exercises. Am J Sports Med 1996;24(4): 518–527.

[78] Bandholm T, Rasmussen L, Aagaard P, et al. Effects of experimental muscle pain on shoulder-abduction force steadiness and muscle activity in healthy subjects. Eur J Appl Physiol 2008;102(6):643–650.

[79] Falla D, Farina D, Dahl MK, et al. Muscle pain induces task-dependent changes in cervical agonist/antagonist activity. J Appl Physiol 2007;102(2): 601–609.

[80] Moseley GL, Nicholas MK, Hodges PW. Does anticipation of back pain predispose to back trouble? Brain 2004;127(Pt 10): 2339–2347.

[81] Moseley GL, Hodges PW. Are the changes in postural control associated with low back pain caused by pain interference? Clin J Pain 2005;21(4):323–329.

[82] Seidler RD. Multiple motor learning experiences enhance motor adaptability. J Cogn Neurosci 2004;16(1):65–73.

[83] Gandevia SC, Refshauge KM, Collins DF. Proprioception: peripheral inputs and perceptual interactions. Adv Exp Med Biol 2002;508:61–68.

[84] Dickson J. Proprioceptive control of human movement. London: Lepus Books; 1974.

[85] Fitzpatrick R, Burke D, Gandevia SC. Task-dependent reflex responses and movement illusions evoked by galvanic vestibular stimulation in standing humans. J Physiol 1994;478(2): 363–372.

[86] Yasuda T, Nakagawa T, Inoue H, et al. The role of the labyrinth, proprioception and plantar

mechanosensors in the maintenance of an upright posture. Eur Arch Otorhinolaryngol 1999;256 (Suppl. 1):S27–S32.

[87] Bergenheim M, Johansson H, Pedersen J, et al. Ensemble coding of muscle stretches in afferent populations containing different types of muscle afferents. Brain Res 1996;734 (1–2):157–166.

[88] Matthews PBC. Muscle spindles: their messages and their fusimotor supply. In: Brookhart JM, Mountcastle VB, Brooks VB, Geiger SR, editors. Handbook of physiology, vol. 2. Bethesda, MD: Motor control. American Physiological Society; 1981 [Chaper 6].

[89] Matthews PBC. Proprioceptors and their contribution to somatosensory mapping: complex messages require complex processing. Can J Physiol Pharmacol 1988;66:430–438.

[90] Miall RC, Ingram HA, Cole JD, Gauthier GM. Weight estimation in a "deafferented" man and in control subjects: are judgements influenced by peripheral or central signals? Exp Brain Res 2000;133(4): 491–500.

[91] Sinclair DC. Cutaneous sensation and the doctrine of specific energy. Brain 1955;78:584–614.

[92] Sorensen KL, Hollands MA, Patla E. The effects of human ankle muscle vibration on posture and balance during adaptive locomotion. Exp Brain Res 2002;143(1):24–34.

[93] Wall PD. Cord cells responding to touch, damage, and temperature of skin. J Neurophysiol 1960;23:197–210.

[94] Wall PD. The somatosensory system. In: Gazzaniga MS, Blackmore C, editors. Handbook of psychobiology. London: Academic Press; 1975.

[95] Ellrich J, Hopf HC. Cerebral potentials are not evoked by activation of Golgi tendon organ afferents in human abductor hallucis muscle. Electromyogr Clin Neurophysiol 1998;38(3): 137–139.

[96] Gardner EP. Somatosensory cortical mechanisms of feature detection in tactile and kinesthetic discrimination. Can J Physiol Pharmacol 1987;66:439–454.

[97] Lemon RN, Porter R. Short-latency peripheral afferent inputs to pyramidal and other neurones in the precentral cortex of conscious monkeys. In: Gordon G, editor. Active touch. Oxford: Pergamon Press; 1978. p. 91–103.

[98] Roland PE. Sensory feedback to the cerebral cortex during voluntary movement in man. Behav Brain Sci 1978;1:129–171.

[99] Bagesteiro LB, Sarlegna FR, Sainburg RL. Differential influence of vision and proprioception on control of movement distance. Exp Brain Res 2006;171(3):358–370.

[100] Bard C, Paillard J, Lajoie Y, et al. Role of afferent information in the timing of motor commands: a comparative study with a deafferented patient. Neuropsychologia 1992;30(2):201–206.

[101] Chernikoff R, Taylor FV. Reaction time to kinesthetic stimulation resulting from sudden arm displacement. J Exp Psychol 1952;43:1–8.

[102] Cockerill IM. The development of ballistic skill movements. In: Whiting HTA, editor. Readings in sports psychology. London: Henry Kimpton; 1972.

[103] Desmedt JE, Godaux E. Ballistic skilled movements: load compensation and patterning of the motor commands. Prog Clinical Neurophysiol 1978;4:21–55.

[104] Lashley KS. The accuracy of movement in the absence of excitation from the moving organ. Am J Physiol 1917;43:169–194.

[105] Taub E. Movement in nonhuman primates deprived of somatosensory feedback. Exerc Sports Sci Rev 1976;4:335–374.

[106] Taub E, Berman AJ. Movement and learning in the absence of sensory feedback. In: Freedman SJ, editor. The neurophysiology of spatially orientated behavior. Homewood, IL: Dorsey Press; 1968.

[107] Bobath B. The application of physiological principles to stroke rehabilitation. Practitioner 1979;223:793–794.

[108] Smith DL, Akhtar AJ, Garraway WM. Proprioception and spatial neglect after stroke. Age Ageing 1983;12(1):63–69.

[109] Azar B. Why can't this man feel whether or not he's standing up? APA Monitor 1998;29(6).

[110] Mulder T, den Otter R, van Engelen B. The regulation of fine movements in patients with Charcot Marie Tooth, type Ia: some ideas about continuous adaptation. Motor Control 2001;5(2):200–214.

[111] Rothwell JC, Traub MM, Day BL, et al. Manual performance in a de-afferented man. Brain 1982;105:515–542.

[112] Jones LA. Motor illusions: what do they reveal about proprioception. Psychol Bull 1988;103(1):72–86.

[113] Burke D, Hagbarth KE, Lofstedt L. Muscle spindle activity in man during shortening and lengthening contractions. J Physiol 1977;277:131–142.

[114] Coggeshall RE, Hong KAHP, Langford LA, et al. Discharge characteristics of fine medial articular afferents at rest and during passive movement of the inflamed knee joints. Brain Res 1983;272:185–188.

[115] Connor NP, Abbs JH. Movement-related skin strain associated with goal-oriented lip actions. Exp Brain Res 1998; 123(3):235–241.

[116] Edin B. Cutaneous afferents provide information about knee joint movements in humans. J Physiol 2001;531(Pt 1): 289–297.

[117] Gandevia SC, McCloskey DI, Burke D. Kinaesthetic signals and muscle contraction. Trends Neurosci 1992;15(2):64–65.

[118] Jenkins DHR. Ligament injuries and their treatment. London: Chapman & Hall Medical; 1985.

[119] Johansson H, Sjolander P, Sojka P. Receptors in the knee

and their role in the biomechanics of the joint. Crit Rev Biomed Eng 1991; 18(5):341–368.

[120] Johansson H, Djupsjobacka M, Sjolander P. Influence on the gamma-muscle spindle system from muscle afferents stimulated by KCl and lactic acid. Neurosci Res 1993; 16(1):49–57.

[121] Krauspe R, Schmidt M, Schaible HG. Sensory innervation of the anterior cruciate ligament. J Bone Joint Surg (A) 1992;74(3):390–397.

[122] Lee J, Ring PA. The effect of local anaesthesia on the appreciation of passive movement in the great toe of man. Proc Physiolog Soc 1954;56–57.

[123] Nielsen J, Pierrot-Deseilligny E. Patterns of cutaneous inhibition of the propriospinal-like excitation to human upper limb motorneurons. J Physiol 1991;434:169–182.

[124] Pedersen J, Sjölander P, Wenngren BI, Johansson H. Increased intramuscular concentration of bradykinin increases the static fusimotor drive to muscle spindles in neck muscles of the cat. Pain 1997; 70(1):83–91.

[125] Ramcharan JE, Wyke B. Articular reflexes at the knee joint: an electromyographic study. Am J Physiol 1972; 223(6):1276–1280.

[126] Schaible HG, Grubb BD. Afferents and spinal mechanisms of joint pain. Pain 1993;55:5–54.

[127] Vallbo AB. Activity from skin mechanoreceptors recorded percutaneously in awake human subjects. Exp Neurol 1968; 21:270–289.

[128] Vallbo AB, Hagbarth KE, Torebjork HE, et al. Somatosensory, proprioceptive and sympathetic activity in human peripheral nerve. Physiolog Rev 1979;59(4): 919–957.

[129] Vallbo AB, Johansson RS. The tactile sensory innervation of the glabrous skin of the human hand. In: Gordon G, editor. Active touch. Oxford: Pergamon Press; 1978. p. 29–54.

[130] Wyke B. The neurology of joints. Ann R Coll Surg Engl 1967; 42:25–50.

[131] Wyke BD. Articular neurology and manipulative therapy. In: Glasgow EF, Twomey LT, Scull ER, Kleynhans AM, Idczek RM, editors. Aspects of manipulative therapy. Edinburgh: Churchill Livingstone; 1985. p. 72–77.

[132] Ginanneschi F, Del Santo F, Dominici F, et al. Changes in corticomotor excitability of hand muscles in relation to static shoulder positions. Exp Brain Res 2005;161(3):374–382.

[133] Eccles JC, Eccles RM, Lundberg A. The convergence of monosynaptic excitatory afferents on the many different species of alpha motoneurons. J Physiol 1957;137:22–50.

[134] Eccles RM, Lundberg A. Integrating patterns of Ia synaptic actions on motoneurones of hip and knee muscles. J Physiol 1958;144:271–298.

[135] Luscher HR, Clamann HP. Relation between structure and function in information transfer in spinal monosynaptic reflex. Physiolog Rev 1992;72(1): 71–99.

[136] Gielen CCAM, Ramaekers L, van Zuylen EJ. Long latency stretch reflexes as co-ordinated functional responses in man. J Physiol 1988;407:275–292.

[137] O'Sullivan MC, Eyre JA, Miller S. Radiation of the phasic stretch reflex in biceps brachii to muscles of the arm in man and its restriction during development. J Physiol 1991;439:529–543.

[138] Baith ID, Harrison PH. Stretch reflexes in human abdominal muscles. Exp Brain Res 2004; 159:206–213.

Motor abilities

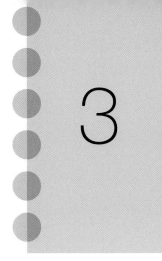

When we observed an individual performing a specific task in which they are talented we often refer to them as being "skilful". Levels of skilfullness can be observed even in normal daily activities such as the unskilled waddle of a toddler in contrast to the skilful walking of an adult. Similarly, we can instantly recognize the dysfunctional "unskilful" gait of a person with an injury.

A skill is how well a person can perform a given task. The proficiency in performing any skill is dependent partly on practice but also on the individual's cognitive, sensory and motor abilities.

Motor abilities are motor control building blocks that underlie all movement.[1,2] To be able to walk it is necessary to have control of balance, multi-limb and whole-body coordination as well as to have control of several other abilities. If any of these abilities is affected the skill of walking will be affected, as well as several other skills that depend on balance and coordination. Some of these specific control losses can be assessed, identified and become the focus of the therapeutic intervention.

In this chapter the different motor abilities are described. Their assessment and specific therapeutic intervention will be discussed in Chapter 12 (see also DVD).

Motor complexity model

The area of motor abilities is extensive and it is estimated that there are numerous such underlying abilities, perhaps running into the hundreds.[3] As they are presented in the literature they are impractical as a model for rehabilitation. I have, therefore, taken the liberty of re-organizing them into a practical clinical approach. As a consequence, some of the abilities' names have been changed to make them user-friendly and new abilities have been added (with apologies to Fleishman).[1,2]

One clinically useful approach is to classify abilities according to their level of motor complexity. In this classification abilities are categorized into four levels, with skill being the top level (Fig. 3.1):
- Parametric abilities
- Synergistic abilities
- Composite abilities
- Skill.

Parametric abilities are the least complex control factors in this model. These abilities can be best described by looking at a simple movement such as reaching. Several variables of this movement can be modified without altering the overall pattern (these are the movement parameters described in Ch. 2). The movement can be executed with varying degrees of force and at different velocities (fast/slow). It can be carried out using different arm lengths (range); with the elbow fully extended or partially flexed. We can repeat this pattern of movement for long or short duration depending on our endurance. From this we can identify four such parametric abilities:
- Force
- Velocity/speed /rate
- Length
- Endurance.

The next level up in complexity is synergistic ability. During the reaching action, elbow flexors

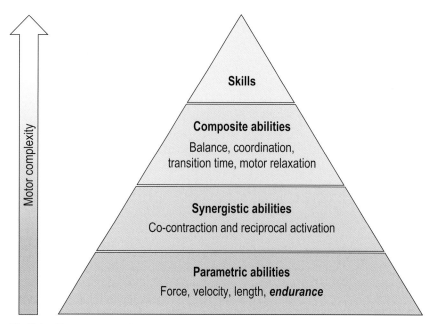

Fig 3.1 ● The motor complexity model presenting some of the important abilities underlying movement control.

and extensors have to be simultaneously controlled. As the movement variables are modified in one group they have to be reflected in the "opposite" group. Hence, *synergistic ability* is about the relationships between muscle groups or between movement pairs (flexion–extension, adduction–abduction, internal–external rotation or any combination of these patterns). There are two identifiable synergistic control patterns:

* Reciprocal activation
* Co-contraction.

Reciprocal activation serves to produce movement while co-contraction increases the stiffness and stability (steadiness) of joints during static posture and movement.[4–7]

Further up the complexity model are the *composite* abilities. These abilities rely on other composite abilities, but also on the less complex parametric and synergistic abilities. Using the arm-reaching movement as an example, it was identified that synergistic ability is needed for elbow movement. However, what happens during simultaneous shoulder and elbow movement? Now, the motor complexity has moved a notch up. The elbow synergistic control has to integrate with that of the shoulder. The harmonious

coupling of the two areas can be considered as *coordination* ability. If at the same time the hand was to manipulate an object, the fine harmonious working of the fingers could be considered as *fine coordination*. The movement of the whole arm is *single-limb coordination* and *multi-limb coordination* if we were synchronously moving the other arm. Since the arms are attached to the rest of the body we have to also consider the harmonious integration of movement between the limbs and the trunk as *body coordination*.

However, there are other factors that come into play while we stand. Upright posture and locomotion depends on body coordination ability, but also on *balance or postural stability*. Furthermore, in daily activity we tend to perform in succession various tasks. The reaching movement, if it were while cooking, would be followed by actions such as holding, whisking or tossing food in a pan, etc. The ability to smoothly and rapidly change between actions is termed here as *transition time*. It is the time it takes to reorganize movement control between two dissimilar events. Finally, if the cooking was for a large number of guests and under a time pressure, we might find that our shoulders are tense and may feel achy and stiff. This psychomotor response to stress will be termed here as *motor relaxation ability*.

From the description above four major composite abilities have been identified:

* Coordination (fine, single- multi-limb and body coordination) ability
* Balance/postural stability
* Transition time
* Relaxation ability.

The individual's skills are placed at the top of the motor complexity model as they contain various combinations of the abilities described above.

Abilities can affect each other, but they can also exist as independent motor losses. For example, in the hand of a stroke patient coordination ability can be affected independently of force and velocity abilities.[8,9]

The classification of abilities by complexity is a useful clinical tool. It provides a rational and methodical approach for assessing and treating specific motor control changes.

Parametric abilities

Force control

Force control is the ability to provide adequate force for optimal execution of movement. It is the ability to regulate force as well as recovering force losses. Included in force control is the ability to fully relax muscles. The way to think about force control is to imagine a light dimmer switch – it can be switched on/off or gradually dimmed.

Force control is the ability to regulate the force rather than make someone stronger. For example, a stroke patient can deliver a bone-crushing handshake, but may not be able to fine grade the squeezing force between low, medium and high forces.[10,11] Conversely, in children with hemiplegia there are force losses but force regulation is saved in the affected hand.[12,13]

Force control is also the ability to fully relax muscles, i.e. no force. During movement some muscle groups will be motorically inactive. This motor relaxation is as important as motor activation for the execution of normal functional movement. The inability to relax force often results in severe movement dysfunction, such as seen in writer's cramp (dystonias) or in stroke patients.[14–17]

Force loss on the other hand is the inability to generate sufficient force for the optimal execution of movement. Force loss can be due to direct physiological and pathological changes to the muscle tissue or its motor innervations. However, the most common manifestation is in failure of voluntary activation seen in musculoskeletal injuries. Like a light dimmer switch, the muscle forces are turned down by the central nervous system (CNS) to unload the damaged or sensitive tissues (Ch. 7).[18–24] Centrally mediated force losses can also be seen in stroke patients as unilateral weakness (hemiparesis) or complete force loss (hemiplegia).[16]

Frequently, force loss is the most obvious movement deficit and can become the unjustified focus of treatment[25,26], sometimes at the expense of overlooking other motor control changes.

Length control

Length control is the ability to effectively regulate the range of movement. This include both the elongation and shortening control of the muscles.

Length control changes are often observed in injury as a narrowing of the ranges of movement. This is a protection strategy to prevent further tissue damage. The hypersensitivity to stretching and reflexive guarding seen after injury is an example of length control. This can be seen during straight-leg raising, where there is a sudden resistance to hip flexion by muscle guarding. Another example is the loss of flexion relaxation of the back muscle in patients with chronic low back pain (CLBP).[27] This is a length protection strategy to prevent the individual from bending fully forward. Regulation of length can be an important issue for patient with damaged CNS. For example, in stroke patient the hypertonic, hyper-flexed wrist and hand partly represent a dysfunctional control of length.

Often in rehabilitation the focus is on achieving maximum length. However, the inability to achieve maximum length could equally be due to an inability to effectively shorten the muscle. This is seen, for example, in neck conditions where there is an inability to rotate the neck to the symptomatic side (even when pain subsides). This could be due to changes in shortening-force control of the neck's rotators. Similarly patients with stiff, non-painful, frozen shoulder may find full flexion difficult even after regaining the passive range of flexion. This may be due to the inability to produce effective length-force shortening of shoulder flexors to elevate the arm (Fig. 3.2). Hence, the therapeutic focus should be on the length-shortening synergy of the movement pairs (see below).

The control of length also relates to the maximum range, i.e. how far an active movement can be executed. Range losses are often seen in musculoskeletal conditions where the patient, due to immobilization or pain, was unable to use the full range of movement. This length change is partly shortening

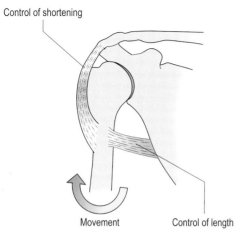

Control of shortening

Movement   Control of length

Fig 3.2 • Active range depends on control of shortening and lengthening of the synergistic pairs.

adaptation in the muscles and connective tissues, but also a dysfunctional "learned shortening" within the neuromuscular continuum.

Length adaptation raises the issue of active and passive flexibility. Active flexibility is the maximum joint range achieved by active shortening and elongation of the local muscles. Passive flexibility is the extreme physiological range of a joint, achieved when all the local muscles are relaxed. If you extend your fingers actively, and without assistance, you will reach a specific range. Keep the fingers in the same position, then using the other hand push the fingers further into extension while relaxing the stretched hand. The passive range should be greater than the active range. Therefore, *passive stretching is useful for improving passive range whereas length control is necessary for active flexibility*. This has important clinical implications. For example, patients with the stiff phase of frozen shoulder can be stretched passively into shoulder flexion. However, when they are instructed to stand and raise their arm, they often can only achieve a relative small degree of flexion – a dysfunctional active range. Passive stretching does not necessarily improve the active range. For improvements in active range the patients should actively move their shoulder at the end ranges (see Ch. 12, Challenging length control and functional stretching).

Velocity/speed control

Speed ability is the capacity to regulate the rate of movement (acceleration/deceleration) and the ability to produce maximum speed of movement.

The ability to regulate the speed is seen, for example, when moving the computer mouse at various speeds to control the screen pointer.

Maximum speed is how fast a movement or a task can be made between two targets. For example, walking a certain distance, reaching for an object or producing an explosive force (mixture of velocity and force). It is also the rate of producing static peak force, such as seen in sudden isometric contraction to block or resist a sudden perturbation.

Changes in speed ability are often seen in musculoskeletal injuries. Individuals tend to slow down their movement as an evasive strategy to pain but also to reduce the forces at the area of damage (reduce the speed = reduce the force).[27–32] For example, patients with lower back pain tend to adapt a slow walk, which may not fully recover even when they are no longer in pain.

Neuromuscular endurance

In the context of motor rehabilitation, endurance is defined as the ability to maintain a physical activity until it can no longer be continued (*neuromuscular fatigue*). Fatigue often manifests as pain, reduced force and velocity of the affected muscles. The symptoms of fatigue are relieved by a period of rest.[33]

A common clinical observation is that individuals with musculoskeletal injuries often demonstrate reduced neuromuscular endurance in the area of damage, even in the absence of pain.[27,34–38] A similar observation is seen in patients who have suffered CNS damage, such as stroke and multiple sclerosis.[39–42] Individuals who suffer from non-traumatic conditions such as trapezius myalgia and chronic neck pain also experience reduced endurance in the painful muscles during repetitive tasks (Ch. 9).[43]

Reduced neuromuscular endurance is associated with central control mechanisms, which are partly reflexive (spinal) and cognitive/psychomotor (higher centres).[33,42,44] It is also partly due to peripheral factors such as muscle atrophy following disuse or immobilization.

Endurance can be improved by physical training and degraded by disuse or injury. It suggests that the central mechanisms that control endurance are mutable and could be influenced by neuromuscular rehabilitation.

Synergistic abilities

Reciprocal activation and co-contraction control

Synergistic control represents the fact that "muscles don't work alone", but in a complex relationship to other muscles.[45] This has important implications for rehabilitation. Damage to one group will inevitably alter the control of all its synergists. Even fatigue or delayed muscle soreness in one muscle group will have an influence on control of the non-exercised synergists. For example, fatigued hamstrings will influence the control of non-exercised quadriceps and similarly fatigued biceps will influence triceps control.[46–48] The effect is likely to spread even to more distant synergists. For example, fatigue in quadriceps will influence the control of the non-exercised gastrocnemius muscle.[49] Hence, it may be more effective to engage the synergistic pairs and whole movement cycles rather than single-muscle or single-direction rehabilitation (e.g. biceps curls).

There are two synergistic control patterns during movement (Box 3.1):

- Reciprocal activation
- Co-contraction.

Reciprocal activation is the simultaneous, active shorting and elongation of muscle pairs needed to produce movement at a joint.

Co-contraction is the simultaneous activation of several muscle groups to stabilize joints during static postures (static stabilization or steadiness) or during movement (dynamic stabilization). Co-contraction also has a role in refining movement. [4,5,50–55]

The two synergistic patterns can be observed, for example, during head rotation. Some muscles will produce the rotation movement (reciprocal activation) while others will dynamically stabilize the head (co-contraction), keeping it upright and preventing it from flopping to the side. Once the head has reached its position, all the neck muscles co-contract statically to maintain the head in the upright position (otherwise the head will fall to the side).

During various motor activities, these patterns of contraction take place jointly but with one pattern being dominant, depending on the task and the angle of the limb (see Box 3.1).[56,57] It should be noted that there are no specific muscles for reciprocal activation or co-contraction. Muscles can switch their roles between being stabilizers or "movers", or both, depending on the position of the limb and the patterns of movement.[57–59]

It has been demonstrated that both patterns of activation have separate cortical control centres, reflecting their distinct functional roles.[60,61] During motor learning, motor control transforms from predominantly co-contractions into more reciprocal patterns (which are more energy-efficient).[62]

Relative factors with synergisms

The two synergistic patterns represent the relationship between several factors that control the movement pairs (Fig. 3.3):

- The relative activation of the parametric abilities
- The relative timing and duration
- Dominance or failure of one of the synergistic patterns.

The relative relationship of parametric abilities can be observed in reciprocal activation. During

> **Box 3.1**
>
> **Home lab**
> Co-contraction and reciprocal activation exercise. With an outstretched arm draw large imaginary numbers from 1 to 10. Focus on your shoulder and feel how the muscles are reciprocally activated. Now draw small-amplitude numbers as fast as possible. You should now feel the shoulder muscles co-contract (as well as the rest of your body).

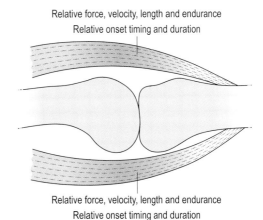

Relative force, velocity, length and endurance
Relative onset timing and duration

Relative force, velocity, length and endurance
Relative onset timing and duration

Fig 3.3 • Synergistic control includes the relative parametric as well as the relative timing and duration in activation of the movement pairs.

rhythmic movement force will increase on one side while reducing on the other; there is muscle elongation on one and shortening on the other. Velocity will be equal on both sides; however, one will be lengthening while the other shortening. In injury and pain conditions this normal relationship is modified. For example, quadriceps inhibition and hamstrings hyperexcitability have been demonstrated in knee injuries.[63–65]

Timing and duration in synergies

Imagine a simple repetitive movement such as elbow flexion–extension. During the phase change (i.e. flexion to extension), the muscles in the movement pairs will have to reverse their action from contraction to relaxation. These changes require complex synchronization in relative timing between the muscle pairs (Fig. 3.4). Furthermore, the relative duration of contraction or relaxation between the synergists also has to be finely synchronized.[32,66–73] Such changes in timing and duration have been demonstrated in patients with lower back pain.[68–71,74–78] There is some

evidence that timing and duration issues may predispose an individual to injury.[79,80]

One aspect of timing that has received much attention in recent years is the *onset time*. This represents the period between the initiation of an action and the relative onset time of different muscles.[32,66–73] This method has been used in research to examine how the onset timing changes in various musculoskeletal injuries and pain conditions.

Dysfunctional synergistic control

Failure in synergistic control can be due to several underlying mechanisms. It can be due to a dysfunctional control of parametric abilities within the synergism, i.e. the relative force, length and velocity. It can be about the relative timing and duration between the movement pairs. Another possibility is that one of the synergistic patterns becomes more dominant or the patient is unable to fully recruit that pattern to produce normal movement.

A change in favour of or dominance of one pattern of synergistic control has been demonstrated in

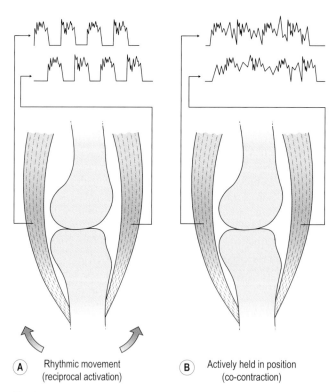

A Rhythmic movement (reciprocal activation)

B Actively held in position (co-contraction)

Fig 3.4 • Electromyograph of synergists during reciprocal activation and co-contraction. **A,** Electromyograph (EMG) trace reciprocal activation. **B,** EMG trace co-contraction.

individuals with intact and damaged motor system. Patients with CLBP tend to increase their co-contraction strategy during movement.[30,81,82] The dominance of co-contraction can also be seen in conditions such as writer's cramp and hypertonicity in stroke patients.[14,17,83–88] In stroke patients this was attributed to malfunction of the centres that control movement synergisms.[61] It is also possible that one of the synergistic patterns becomes less effectively controlled. For example, functional instability of the ankle is associated with co-contraction failure.[89] The loss of normal swinging of the affected arm in stroke could be seen as the inability to control reciprocal activation.

Composite abilities

The composite abilities described below have been narrowed down and modified to the ones that I feel are clinically important. Composite abilities are influenced not only by other abilities in the group but also by the contraction and synergistic abilities (Fig. 3.5).

Coordination

Coordination is the harmonious and synchronous control of two or more joints or body masses. Coordination may be affected locally, in the hand following immobilization (fine cordination);[90] more widely, in the movement of a whole limb (single-limb coordination); bilaterally, in the coordinated activities of limbs (multi-limb coordination) or extensively, affecting the whole body (whole-body coordination).

Generally, patients with CNS conditions are more likely to have extensive coordination losses. In musculoskeletal conditions coordination losses may be more localized, pertaining to the area of damage or pain.[9,90,91]

Balance

Balance is the ability to efficiently maintain upright movement or stance with minimal physical stress and expenditure of energy. This ability depends on several factors: the sensory inputs from the vestibular apparatus, vision,[92] proprioception, hearing,[93,94] central integration/processing of sensory information[95] and control of whole-body coordination and balance.[3] Failure in any of these systems or processes will manifest as unsteadiness and unrefined movement and stance or, at worst, the inability to maintain an upright posture.

There are differences between static balance (standing still, sitting) and dynamic balance (walking, running and climbing stairs). Dynamic balance is more complex as it makes greater demands on motor control and cognitive-motor processes. Patients who

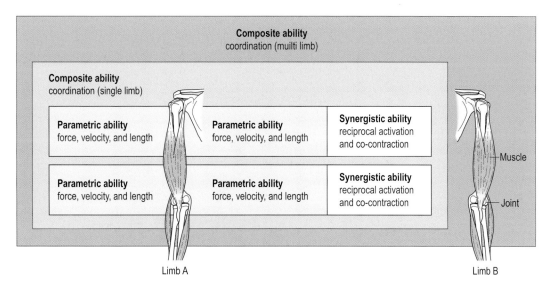

Fig 3.5 • Motor abilities in control of a single and two limbs. At the lower end of the motor complexity are the parametric abilities of the individual muscle groups. Next, is the relative paired activation of the muscle groups at synergistic level. The composite ability incorporates the underlying parametric and synergistic abilities.

demonstrate balance losses should be challenged both in dynamic and static balance (Ch. 12).

Postural stability and instability

Postural stability relates to local proprioception or motor control losses from the lower limbs or the trunk/neck that affect balance. It is often measured as the magnitude of sway or steadiness to perturbation during standing.

In musculoskeletal injuries reduced proprioception or loss of normal control of synergism at the area of damage may produce what seems like a balance loss. For example, patients with lower back pain may display postural instability associated with delayed response times in the trunk muscle.[68–71,75,76] Similarly, patients with an ankle injury may find balancing difficult on the injured side due to proprioceptive and synergistic control changes in the lower limb.[96]

This is somewhat different to central losses where balance is more widely affected. In these conditions the patient may find balance to be equally difficult on each or both legs, or even whilst sitting.

The distinction between balance and postural stability has some clinical implications. In musculoskeletal conditions the losses relate more to postural stability rather than true balance control. Postural instability is more localized (e.g. affecting balance on one limb); patients take less time to recover and may use compensatory sensory-motor strategies that overcome these losses (weight-bearing on the non-affected side). However, central or vestibular causes for balance losses are generally more extensive conditions, require longer recovery periods and may only partially recover depending on the extent of central damage.

Transition time

Transition time is the period it takes to reorganize movement between two dissimilar events and to carry out the subsequent task skilfully (Fig. 3.6). For example, if you hop on a single leg from side to side and than suddenly stop, the body will sway until it settles into the static balance. This represents the organization time between dynamic and static balance. If this is repeated several times you will find that the organization of the static balance becomes progressively and more rapidly controlled.

Transition rate represents the duration it takes for sensory inputs to reach central motor areas, to process this information, to make decision

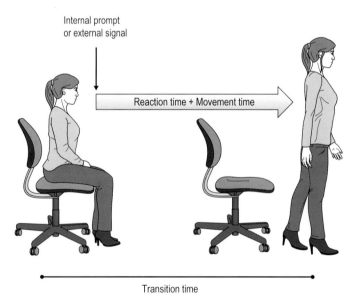

Internal prompt or external signal

Reaction time + Movement time

Transition time

Fig 3.6 • Transition time is the total period needed to organize and execute one task after another.

about the action to take and the time it takes the motor commands to reach the muscles (reaction time). It also includes the period required to complete all the postural adjustments and the observable execution of the movement in the subsequent task (movement time). The different elements within this chain of events can occur within a fraction of a second, too rapidly to be assessed separately in the absence of lab tools. Therefore, the term "transition time" has been introduced as a clinical reality. What is humanly possible (in my experience) is to observe the grand total of how rapidly and smoothly a person can change between two activities – inaccurate, but good enough clinically.

Longer organization times can be often observed in various musculoskeletal injuries and in patients with central damage.[28–32,97] A stroke patient may have difficulties in organization within or between tasks, such as sitting, getting up and walking, or walking and turning around. Such activities are marked with a long pause for reorganization between the two actions.

Interestingly in sports, some triathletes report discoordination when running after cycling. This was associated with the inability of the motor system to effectively reorganize itself between the two intense physical activities.[98]

Motor relaxation

Motor relaxation is the ability to reduce neuromuscular activity to the optimal level necessary for maintaining a motor task or to become inactive. Motor relaxation represents the flip side of motor activation. It is paradoxically a neurologically active motor process.

Motor relaxation and force relaxation control (see force ability) are seen in different conditions. There are several conditions where the individual develops pain conditions by tension holding, such as trapezius myalgia or chronic neck pain (Ch. 9). It is the inability to relax in a psycho-motor dimension. Force relaxation ability, on the other hand, is associated with more reflexive mechanisms where specific areas become hypertonic such as seen in central nervous system damage.

Although motor relaxation and force ability are the outcome of different processes, the clinical management has the same aims (relax the overactive muscles) using the same approach (motor relaxation).

Mutability of abilities

According to motor control research, some of the motor abilities described above are a mixture of genetic traits and learning that develop during childhood and adolescence.[1–3] Coordination, for example, is one such ability that is genetically determined.[99] Once the motor system has matured in adult life some of these abilities become resistant to change. However, they may retain a limited capacity to be modified by practice.[100,101] In other words each individual has a "personal best" in any of these control variables (except in the parametric and synergistic abilities that rely partly on central and peripheral adaptation to training).

The aim in neuromuscular re-abilitation is to help the person recover their losses to the "best of their ability", rather than improving their personal best. It has been demonstrated consistently that all abilities in the motor complexity model can be affected by musculoskeletal injury, psychomotor conditions or CNS damage, see summary in Table 3.1.

It should be noted that in musculoskeletal conditions there are no single ability changes. They are part of an overall protective strategy, with multiple options and containing a variety of component changes (the abilities). One common misconception about abilities is to view them as a unique, single outcome (or cause) of a particular condition. This is exemplified by the core stability training approach, where the focus is on normalizing the timing delay in the abdominal muscles. However, this change is only a small element in the overall motor strategy of a person suffering from back pain, as depicted in Table 3.1.

Can motor abilities be normalized?

There is some evidence that motor abilities can be normalized by training and rehabilitation.

Most obvious changes can be observed in the parametric abilities. For example, physical training has been shown to reduce arthrogenic inhibition in the knee (force control).[23,169,170] In patients with early osteoarthritis of the knees and post meniscectomy, exercise rehabilitation has been shown to improve force and endurance abilities.[169,171] In chronic lower back patients lumbar extension exercises were shown to improve trunk muscle strength, cross-sectional

Table 3.1 Examples of motor abilities affected in various conditions

Conditions	Parametric motor abilities				Synergistic		Composite		
	Force	Length	Velocity	Endurance	Co-contraction/ reciprocal activation	Coordination	Balance/postural stability	Transition time	Relaxation
Lower back pain	Force losses in trunk muscles in acute and chronic lower back pain (CLBP) patients.[18,19,37,102,103]	Loss of flexion relaxation in the spinal muscles during flexion in patients with CLBP. Extensors activation prevents full forward bending.[27] Individuals with high pain-related fear had smaller excursions of the lumbar spine for reaches to all targets at 3 and 6 weeks, but not at 12 weeks following pain onset.[31] Smaller stride length.[30]	Reduced velocity of trunk movement during flexion induced back pain.[32] Individuals with high pain-related fear had smaller peak velocities and accelerations of the lumbar spine and hip joints, even after resolution of back pain.[31] Walking velocity significantly lower in lower back pain (LBP) patients.[28-30]	Increased fatigability of trunk muscles in patients with CLBP.[27,36-38]	Impaired postural control of the lumbar spine is associated with delayed trunk/ abdominal muscles response times in CLBP patients.[68-71,74-78] Increase in trunk co-contraction in CLBP patients.[79,82] Increase co-contraction in trunk during walking and additional cognitive demands.[30]	Lumbar spine-hip joint coordination altered in back pain subjects.[148] Dis-coordination in pelvis-thorax coordination in LBP.[28,29]	Changes in postural control in CLBP.[72,158] Impaired postural control of the lumbar spine associated with delayed muscle response times in CLBP patients.[76] Changes in postural control unrelated to pain in CLBP.[159] Post spinal surgery postural control changes both in pain and pain-free subjects. However, more evident in the symptomatic subjects.[160] Hip strategy for balance control in quiet standing is affected in CLBP.[161] Experimental muscle pain changes feedforward postural responses of the trunk muscles.[68]	Compared to healthy controls, persons with LBP exhibited a reduced ability to adapt trunk–pelvis coordination and spinal muscle activity to sudden changes in walking velocity.[28,29] Slower reaction time in LBP patients. Demonstrated recovery of reaction time with training.[164]	Not studied (but should be).

Conditions	Parametric motor abilities				Synergistic		Composite		
	Force	Length	Velocity	Endurance	Co-contraction/ reciprocal activation	Coordination	Balance/postural stability	Transition time	Relaxation
Non-traumatic chronic. chronic neck pain. Trapezius myalgia. Tension headaches. Traumatic: chronic whiplash.	Demonstrated muscle weakness in cervical muscle in chronic whiplash patients.[104,105] Trapezius myalgia – reduced force in affected side.[106]	Reduced cervical range of motion in whiplash patients and chronic neck pain.[112,113]	Only small non-significant changes in velocity changes in head movement.[119] Longer time to produce peak force for whiplash subjects.[120]	Reduced cervical flexor endurance following whiplash injury.[35] Reduced endurance in neck muscles in chronic.[127] Tension headache – reduced endurance in neck flexors[128]	Changes in synergists' recruitment during isometric (co-contraction) and dynamic (reciprocal activation) in acute whiplash patients.[133] Tension headache – abnormal co-contraction and reciprocal activation in neck muscles.[134,135]	Less refined neck movement in chronic neck pain patients.[113,119] Balance most unstable during gait involving task-specific head movements.[149] Dis-coordinated movement of jaw and head movement in whiplash.[150] Chronic neck pain – abnormal cervical muscle recruitment during coordination exercise.[108,151,152]	Chronic neck pain patients have reduced whole body and head postural stability.[149,162] Tension headache – reduced postural control.[163]	Chronic neck pain patients have reduced head stability during perturbations.[162]	Inability to relax in whiplash, trapezius myalgia and chronic neck pain.[148,149,166] Trapezius myalgia – inability to relax specific muscles.[167] Chronic neck pain – inability to relax different muscles in the neck and shoulder.[151,152,168]

Continued

Table 3.1 Examples of motor abilities affected in various conditions—Cont'd

Conditions	Parametric motor abilities				Synergistic		Composite		
	Force	Length	Velocity	Endurance	Co-contraction/ reciprocal activation	Coordination	Balance/postural stability	Transition time	Relaxation
Knee	Abnormal relationship in force between quadriceps and hamstrings in anterior cruciate ligament (ACL) deficient knee.[63–65] Force losses in quadriceps femoris after ACL repair.[107]	Reduced knee range of motion – external-flexion moment during various gait activities in ACL deficient knees.[64,114–116]	Reduced walking velocity in painful osteoarthritis (OA) knees.[121–123]	Normal endurance in quadriceps pre and post-operative ACL, but forces losses were present.[129,130] ACL damage – increase fatigability of hamstrings during walking.[131]	Two different adaptive strategies following ACL tear. Change in reciprocal and co-contraction strategies.[136] Changes in the timing and duration of knee synergists during movements in ACL tears.[137–139] Reduced stabilization in individuals who have knee instability following ACL rupture with return to pre-injury activities[140] ACL injury – "non-copers" utilize a stabilization strategy which not only is unsuccessful but may lead to excessive joint contact forces and which have the potential to damage articular structures (Rudolph et al 1998). Increase co-contraction during walking in medial OA.[142]	ACL damage. Changes in interjoint coordination of lower limb.[91]	ACL-deficient subjects cannot adequately perform postural adjustments.[182]	Loss of ability to respond normally to sudden postural perturbations in ACL tears. Also non-injured side affected.[182]	Not applicable.

30

Conditions	Parametric motor abilities				Synergistic		Composite		
	Force	Length	Velocity	Endurance	Co-contraction/ reciprocal activation	Coordination	Balance/postural stability	Transition time	Relaxation
Shoulder conditions	Impingement – force deficits and muscular imbalance in the scapular muscles.[108,109] Force control affected (ability to maintain a steady force) during submaximal contraction ~35% MVC.[34]	Although range is reduced, may be associated with pathological changes in tissues.	Impingement – bilateral (painful and non-painful sides) decrease in the time to peak tension during medial rotation of shoulder.[97]	Frozen shoulder- reduced endurance in deltoid.[132] Impingement – reduced endurance of trapezius, deltoideus, infraspiratus, and supraspinatus during submaximal contraction, not related to pain.[34]	Impingement – change in onset timing of rotator cuff muscles during shoulder external rotation in throwers with and without symptoms.[80] Muscular imbalance in the scapular muscles.[108,143] Abnormal muscle recruitment timing in the trapezius and scapular muscle.[144] Abnormal muscle recruitment in the shoulder in symptomatic and asymptomatic subjects, but greater deficits in symptomatic.[145] Frozen shoulder – changes in coordination of different part of trapezius.[146]	No available data.	Not applicable.	No available data.	Not studied

Continued

Table 3.1 Examples of motor abilities affected in various conditions—Cont'd

Conditions	Parametric motor abilities				Synergistic		Composite		
	Force	Length	Velocity	Endurance	Co-contraction/ reciprocal activation	Coordination	Balance/postural stability	Transition time	Relaxation
CNS damage	Stroke – weakness in grip strength and isometric extension.[110,111] Excessive abnormal flexor force limiting voluntary finger extension.[110] Children with hemiplegia – force losses but saved force regulation in affected hand.[12,13]	Stroke – abnormal constraints in range.[117] Abnormal constraints in linkage between activation of the elbow flexors and shoulder extensors, abductors, and external rotators.[118]	Loss of velocity but not timing in ankle movement in incomplete spinal cord injury.[124] Stroke – patients moved their heads at lower velocities.[125] Slower movement velocity.[126]	Fatigability in individuals suffering from a variety of central nervous system (CNS) conditions.[42]	Dysfunctional co-contraction in leg muscles of children with cerebral palsy.[147] Deficits in the coordination of agonist and antagonist muscles in stroke patients.[57,87] Stroke – presence of abnormally large silent duration in co-contraction at different angles. This was correlated with postural instability and oscillations about the final position of the arm after unloading.[57,87]	Stroke – single-limb dis-coordination.[153,154] Change in inter-limb coordination.[154] Discoordination of normal rhythm of swinging the arms.[156] Loss of fine coordination (fine control) in the hand.[157]	Stroke – patients had altered postural adjustments to voluntary head motions during standing.[125]	Increase in time to organize multi-limb coordination at onset of movement. Improves towards the end of movement.[165]	Not studied.

area and endurance.[172–175] In patients with chronic neck pain, endurance and muscle strength improved after 2 weeks' training specific to these abilities.[176] A functional rehabilitation program was shown to improve the velocity of movement ability in lower back and knee damage patients.[164,177]

The synergistic muscle activity in patients with different joint conditions has also been shown to be altered by physical therapy. In functional instability of the ankle, treatment by challenging postural stability virtually eliminated the symptoms of instability as well as significantly changing muscle onset times.[96,178] Similarly, training was shown to change various factors in synergistic control of normal and anterior cruciate ligament (ACL) deficient knees.[179,180] Postural stability and control of coordination was also shown to be improved by TaiChi, which is a movement approach that challenges these motor abilities.[181]

Summary points

- Skill is the measurement of how proficient a person is in performing a particular task.
- Skills depends on a mixture of sensory-motor and cognitive abilities of the individual.
- Motor abilities are the various control factors that underlie movement.
- Motor abilities can be classified according to their level of motor complexity: parametric, synergistic and composite abilities.
- Parametric abilities are: force, velocity/speed/rate, length, endurance.
- There are two identifiable synergistic control patterns: reciprocal activation and co-contraction.
- Reciprocal activation serves to produce movement while co-contraction's role is to increase the stiffness and stability (steadiness) of joints during static posture and movement.
- Composite abilities are: coordination (fine, single- and multi-limb and body coordination), balance/postural stability, transition time and relaxation ability.
- Motor ability changes can be observed in musculoskeletal injuries and pain conditions, and in patients suffering from CNS damage.
- There is some evidence that motor abilities can be normalized by activities that challenge them specifically.

References

[1] Fleishman EA. The structure and measurement of physical fitness. Prentice Hall, NJ: Engelwood Cliffs; 1964.

[2] Fleishman EA. Human abilities and the acquisition of skills. In: Bilodeau EA, editor. Acquisition of skill. New York: Academic Press; 1966.

[3] Schmidt RA, Lee TD. Motor control and learning. 4th ed. UK: Human Kinetics; 2005.

[4] Doemges F, Rack PMH. Changes in the stretch reflex of the human first interosseous muscle during different tasks. J Physiol 1992;447:563–573.

[5] Doemges F, Rack PMH. Task-dependent changes in the response of human wrist joints to mechanical disturbance. J Physiol 1992;447:575–585.

[6] Markolf KL, Graff-Radford A, Amstutz H. In vivo knee stability. A quantitative assessment using an instrumental clinical testing apparatus. J Bone Joint Surg (A) 1979;60:664–674.

[7] Panjabi MM. The stabilizing system of the spine. Part 1. Function, dysfunction, adaptation, and enhancement. J Spinal Dis 1992;5(4):383–389.

[8] Ada L, Canning C, Dwyer T. Effect of muscle length on strength and dexterity after stroke. Clin Rehabil 2000;14(1):55–61.

[9] Canning CG, Ada L, O'Dwyer NJ. Abnormal muscle activation characteristics associated with loss of dexterity after stroke. J Neurol Sci 2000;176(1):45–56.

[10] Fellows SJ, Noth J, Schwarz M. Precision grip and Parkinson's disease. Brain 1998;121(Pt 9):1771–1784.

[11] Raghavan P, Krakauer JW, Gordon AM. Impaired anticipatory control of fingertip forces in patients with a pure motor or sensorimotor lacunar syndrome. Brain 2006;129(Pt 6):1415–1425.

[12] Rameckers EA, Smits-Engelsman BC, Duysens J. Children with spastic hemiplegia are equally able as controls in maintaining a precise percentage of maximum force without visually monitoring their performance. Neuropsychologia 2005;43(13):1938–1945.

[13] Smits-Engelsman BC, Rameckers EA, Duysens J. Muscle force generation and force control of finger movements in children with spastic hemiplegia during isometric tasks. Dev Med Child Neurol 2005;47(5):337–342.

[14] Preibisch C, Berg D, Hofmann E, et al. Cerebral activation patterns in patients with writer's cramp: a

functional magnetic resonance imaging study. J Neurol 2001; 248(1):10–17.

[15] Prodoehl J, MacKinnon CD, Comella CL, et al. Strength deficits in primary focal hand dystonia. Mov Disord 2006; 21(1):18–27.

[16] Winstein C, Wing AM, Whitall, J Motor control and learning principles for rehabilitation of upper limb movement after brain injury. In: Grafman J, Robertson IH, editors. Handbook of neuropsychology, 2nd ed. vol. 9. London: Elsevier; 2003.

[17] Yazawa S, Ikeda A, Kaji R, et al. Abnormal cortical processing of voluntary muscle relaxation in patients with focal hand dystonia studied by movement-related potentials. Brain 1999;122(Pt 7): 1357–1366.

[18] Hides JA, Stokes MJ, Saide M, et al. Evidence of lumbar multifidus muscle wasting ipsilateral to symptoms in patients with acute/subacute low back pain. Spine 1994; 19(2):165–172.

[19] Hides JA, Richardson CA, Jull GA. Multifidus muscle recovery is not automatic after resolution of acute, first-episode low back pain. Spine 1996; 21(23):2763–2769.

[20] Hurley MV, O'Flanagan SJ, Newham DJ. Isokinetic and isometric muscle strength and inhibition after elbow arthroplasty. J Ortho Rheumatol 1991;4:83–95.

[21] Jones DW, Jones DA, Newham DJ. Chronic knee effusion and aspiration: the effect on quadriceps inhibition. Br J Rheumatol 1987;26:370–374.

[22] Spencer JD, Hayes KC, Alexander IJ. Knee joint effusion and quadriceps reflex inhibition in man. Arch Phys Med Rehabil 1984;65:171–177.

[23] Stokes M, Young A. The contribution of reflex inhibition to arthrogenous muscle weakness. Clin Sci 1984;67:7–14.

[24] Ylinen J, Takala EP, Kautiainen H. Association of neck pain, disability and neck pain during maximal effort with neck muscle strength and range of movement in women with chronic non-specific neck pain. Eur J Pain 2004;8(5):473–478.

[25] Mizner RL, Kawaguchi JK, Chmielewski TL. Muscle strength in the lower extremity does not predict postinstruction improvements in the landing patterns of female athletes. J Orthop Sports Phys Ther 2008;38(6):353–361.

[26] Sullivan KJ, Brown DA, Klassen T, et al. Effects of task-specific locomotor and strength training in adults who were ambulatory after stroke: results of the STEPS randomized clinical trial. Phys Ther 2007;87 (12):1580–1602; discussion 1603–1607.

[27] Shirado O, Ito T, Kaneda K, Strax TE. Flexion-relaxation phenomenon in the back muscles. A comparative study between healthy subjects and patients with chronic low back pain. Am J Phys Med Rehabil 1995;74 (2):139–144.

[28] Lamoth CJ, Daffertshofer A, Meijer OG, et al. How do persons with chronic low back pain speed up and slow down? Trunk-pelvis coordination and lumbar erector spinae activity during gait. Gait Posture 2006;23(2):230–239.

[29] Lamoth CJ, Meijer OG, Daffertshofer A, et al. Effects of chronic low back pain on trunk coordination and back muscle activity during walking: changes in motor control. Eur Spine J 2006;15(1):23–40.

[30] Lamoth CJ, Stins JF, Pont M, et al. Effects of attention on the control of locomotion in individuals with chronic low back pain. J Neuroeng Rehabil 2008;5:13.

[31] Thomas JS, France CR, Lavender SA, et al. Effects of fear of movement on spine velocity and acceleration after recovery from low back pain. Spine 2008;33(5):564–570.

[32] Zedka M, Prochazka A, Knight B, et al. Voluntary and reflex control of human back muscles during induced pain. J Physiol 1999;520 (Pt 2):591–604.

[33] Gandevia SC. Spinal and supraspinal factors in human muscle fatigue. Physiol Rev 2001;81(4):1725–1789.

[34] Bandholm T, Rasmussen L, Aagaard P, et al. Force steadiness, muscle activity, and maximal muscle strength in subjects with subacromial impingement syndrome. Muscle Nerve 2006;34 (5):631–639.

[35] Kumbhare DA. Measurement of cervical flexor endurance following whiplash. Disabil Rehabil 2005;27(14):801–807.

[36] Roy SH, De Luca CJ, Casavant DA. Lumbar muscle fatigue and chronic lower back pain. Spine 1989;14(9): 992–1001.

[37] Shirado O, Ito T, Kaneda K, Strax TE. Concentric and eccentric strength of trunk muscles: influence of test postures on strength and characteristics of patients with chronic low-back pain. Arch Phys Med Rehabil 1995;76 (7):604–611.

[38] Suter E, Lindsay D. Back muscle fatigability is associated with knee extensor inhibition in subjects with low back pain. Spine 2001;26(16):E361–E366.

[39] Newham DJ, Davies JM, Mayston MJ. Voluntary force generation and activation in the knee muscles of stroke patients with mild spastic hemiparesis. J Physiol (Lond) 1995;483:128P.

[40] Sheean GL, Murray NM, Rothwell JC, et al. An electrophysiological study of the mechanism of fatigue in multiple sclerosis. Brain 1997;120(Pt 2): 299–315.

[41] Thickbroom GW, Sacco P, Kermode AG, et al. Central motor drive and perception of effort during fatigue in multiple sclerosis. J Neurol 2006;253(8): 1048–1053.

[42] Zwarts MJ, Bleijenberg G, van Engelen BG. Clinical neurophysiology of fatigue. Clin Neurophysiol 2008;119(1):2–10.

[43] Rosendale L, Larsson B, Kristiansen J, et al. Increase in muscle nociceptive substances and anaerobic metabolism in patients with trapezius myalgia: microdialysis in rest and during exercise. Pain 2004;112:324–334.

[44] Benwell NM, Sacco P, Hammond GR, et al. Short-interval cortical inhibition and corticomotor excitability with fatiguing hand exercise: a central adaptation to fatigue? Exp Brain Res 2006;170(2):191–198.

[45] Hughlings Jackson J. On the comparative study of disease of the nervous system. Br Med J 1889;17:355–362.

[46] Maynard J, Ebben WP. The effects of antagonist prefatigue on agonist torque and electromyography. J Strength Cond Res 2003;17(3):469–474.

[47] Semmler JG, Tucker KJ, Allen TJ, et al. Eccentric exercise increases EMG amplitude and force fluctuations during submaximal contractions of elbow flexor muscles. J Appl Physiol 2007;103(3):979–989.

[48] Weir JP, Keefe DA, Eaton JF, et al. Effect of fatigue on hamstring coactivation during isokinetic knee extensions. Eur J Appl Physiol Occup Physiol 1998;78(6):555–559.

[49] Nyland JA, Caborn DN, Shapiro R. Fatigue after eccentric quadriceps femoris work produces earlier gastrocnemius and delayed quadriceps femoris activation during crossover cutting among normal athletic women. Knee Surg Sports Traumatol Arthrosc 1997; 5(3):162–167.

[50] Aagaard P, Simonsen EB, Andersen JL, Magnusson SP, Bojsen-Møller F, Dyhre-Poulsen P. Antagonist muscle coactivation during isokinetic knee extension. Scand J Med Sci Sports 2000;10(2):58–67.

[51] Granata KP, Marras WS. Cost-benefit of muscle cocontraction in protecting against spinal instability. Spine 2000; 25(11):1398–1404.

[52] Gribble PL, Mullin LI, Cothros N, et al. Role of cocontraction in arm movement accuracy. J Neurophysiol 2003; 89(5):2396–2405.

[53] Labriola JE, Lee TQ, Debski RE, et al. Stability and instability of the glenohumeral joint: the role of shoulder muscles. J Shoulder Elbow Surg 2005;14(Suppl. 1): 32S–38S.

[54] van Dieen JH, Kingma I, van der Bug JCE. Evidence for a role of antagonistic cocontraction in controlling trunk stiffness during lifting. J Biomech 2003;36:1829–1836.

[55] Yanagawa T, Goodwin CJ, Shelburne KB, et al. Contributions of the individual muscles of the shoulder to glenohumeral joint stability during abduction. J Biomech Eng 2008;130(2): 021024.

[56] Hodges PW, Gurfinkel VS, Brumagne S, et al. Coexistence of stability and mobility in postural control: evidence from postural compensation for respiration. Exp Brain Res 2002;144(3):293–302.

[57] Levin MF, Dimov M. Spatial zones for muscle coactivation and the control of postural stability. Brain Res 1997;757(1):43–59.

[58] Anderson FC, Pandy MG. Individual muscle contributions to support in normal walking. Gait Posture 2003;17 (2):159–169.

[59] McGill SM, Grenier S, Kaycic N, et al. Coordination of muscle activity to assure stability of the lumber spine. J Electromyogr Kinesiol 2003;13(4):353–359.

[60] Bennett DJ, Gorassini M, Prochazka A. Catching a ball: contribution of intrinsic muscle stiffness, reflexes, and higher order responses. Can J Physiol Pharmacol 1994;72(2):525–534.

[61] Humphrey DR, Reed DJ. Separate cortical systems for control of joint movement and joint stiffness: reciprocal activation and coactivation of antagonist muscles. Adv Neurol 1983;39:347–372.

[62] Lay BS, Sparrow WA, Hughes KM, et al. Practice effects on coordination and control, metabolic energy expenditure, and muscle activation. Hum Move Sci 2002;21(5–6):807–830.

[63] Hole CD, Smit GH, Hammond J, et al. Dynamic control and conventional strength ratios of the quadriceps and hamstrings in subjects with anterior cruciate ligament deficiency. Ergonomics 2000;43(10):1603–1609.

[64] Patel RR, Hurwitz DE, Bush-Joseph CA, et al. Comparison of clinical and dynamic knee function in patients with anterior cruciate ligament deficiency. Am J Sports Med 2003;31(1):68–74.

[65] St Clair Gibson A, Lambert MI, Durandt JJ, et al. Quadriceps and hamstrings peak torque ratio changes in persons with chronic anterior cruciate ligament deficiency. J Orthop Sports Phys Ther 2000;30(7):418–427.

[66] Bonfim TR, Jansen Paccola CA, Barela JA. Proprioceptive and behavior impairments in individuals with anterior cruciate ligament reconstructed knees. Arch Phys Med Rehabil 2003;84:1217–1223.

[67] Hodges PW, Gandevia SC, Richardson CA. Contractions of specific abdominal muscles in postural tasks are affected by respiratory maneuvers. J Appl Physiol 1997;83(3): 753–760.

[68] Hodges PW, Moseley GL, Gabrielsson A, Gandevia SC. Experimental muscle pain changes feedforward postural responses of the trunk muscles. Exp Brain Res 2003;151(2): 262–271.

[69] Hodges PW, Richardson CA. Inefficient muscular stabilization of the lumbar spine associated with low back pain. A motor control evaluation of transversus abdominis. Spine 1996;21(22): 2640–2650.

[70] Hodges PW, Richardson CA. Delayed postural contraction of transversus abdominis in low back pain associated with movement of the lower limb. Spinal Disord 1998;11(1):46–56.

[71] Hodges PW, Richardson CA. Altered trunk muscle recruitment in people with low back pain with upper limb movement at different speeds. Arch Phys Med Rehabil 1999;80(9):1005–1012.

[72] Leinonen V, Kankaanpaa M, Luukkonen M, et al. Disc herniation-related back pain impairs feed-forward control of paraspinal muscles. Spine 2001;26(16): E367–E372.

[73] Madeleine P, Voigt M, Arendt-Nielsen L. Reorganisation of human step initiation during acute experimental muscle pain. Gait Posture 1999;10 (3):240–247.

[74] MacDonald DA, Moseley GL, Hodges PW. The lumbar multifidus: Does the evidence support clinical beliefs? Man Ther 2006;11(4):254–2563 [Epub 2006 May 23].

[75] O'Sullivan P, Twomey L, Allison G, et al. Altered patterns of abdominal muscle activation in patients with chronic low back pain. Aust J Physiother 1997; 43(2):91–98.

[76] Radebold A, Cholewicki J, Polzhofer GK, Greene HS. Impaired postural control of the lumbar spine is associated with delayed muscle response times in patients with chronic idiopathic low back pain. Spine 2001;26(7): 724–730.

[77] Thomas JS, France CR, Sha D, et al. The effect of chronic low back pain on trunk muscle activations in target reaching movements with various loads. Spine 2007;32(26):E801–E808.

[78] Thomas JS, France CR. Pain-related fear is associated with avoidance of spinal motion during recovery from low back pain. Spine 2007;32(16):E460–E466.

[79] Cholewicki J, Silfies SP, Shah RA, et al. Delayed trunk muscle reflex responses increase the risk of low back injuries. Spine 2005;30(23):2614–2620.

[80] Hess SA, Richardson C, Darnell R, Friis P, Lisle D, Myers P. Timing of rotator cuff activation during shoulder external rotation in throwers with and without symptoms of pain. J Orthop Sports Phys Ther 2005;35(12):812–820.

[81] Cholewicki J, Panjabi MM, Khachatryan A. Stabilizing function of trunk flexor-extensor muscles around a neutral spine posture. Spine 1997;22(19):2207–2212.

[82] van Dieen JH, Cholewicki J, Radebold A. Trunk muscle recruitment patterns in patients with low back pain enhance the stability of the lumbar spine. Spine 2003;28(8):834–841.

[83] Chen R, Wassermann EM, Canos M, et al. Impaired inhibition in writer's cramp during voluntary muscle activation. Neurology 1997;49 (4):1054–1059.

[84] Farmer SF, Sheean GL, Mayston MJ, et al. Abnormal motor unit synchronization of antagonist muscles underlies pathological co-contraction in upper limb dystonia. Brain 1998;121(Pt 5):801–814.

[85] Hidler JM, Carroll M, Federovich EH. Strength and coordination in the paretic leg of individuals following acute stroke. IEEE Trans Neural Syst Rehabil Eng 2007;15(4):526–534.

[86] Hughes M, McLellan DL. Increased co-activation of the upper limb muscles in writer's cramp. J Neurol Neurosurg Psychiatry 1985;48(8):782–787.

[87] Levin MF, Selles RW, Verheul MH, Meijer OG. Deficits in the coordination of agonist and antagonist muscles in stroke patients: implications for normal motor control. Brain Res 2000; 853(2):352–369.

[88] Odergren T, Iwasaki N, Borg J, et al. Impaired sensory–motor integration during grasping in writer's cramp. Brain 1996; 119(Pt 2):569–583.

[89] Richie Jr DH. Functional instability of the ankle and the role of neuromuscular control: a comprehensive review. J Foot Ankle Surg 2001;40(4):240–251.

[90] de Jong BM, Coert JH, Stenekes MW, et al. Cerebral reorganisation of human hand movement following dynamic immobilisation. Neuroreport 2003;14(13):1693–1696.

[91] St-Onge N, Duval N, Yahia L, et al. Interjoint coordination in lower limbs in patients with a rupture of the anterior cruciate ligament of the knee joint. Knee Surg Sports Traumatol Arthrosc 2004;12(3):203–216.

[92] Lee DN, Aronson E. Visual proprioceptive control of standing in human infants. Percept Psychophys 1974;15:527–532.

[93] Ashmead DH, Davis DL, Northington A. Contribution of listeners' approaching motion to auditory distance perception. J Exp Psychol Hum Percept Perform 1995;21(2):239–256.

[94] Ashmead DH, Wall RS. Auditory perception of walls via spectral variations in the ambient sound field. J Rehabil Res Dev 1999;36(4):313–322.

[95] Lajoie Y, Teasdale N, Bard C, Fleury M. Attentional demands for static and dynamic equilibrium. Exp Brain Res 1993;97:139–144.

[96] Freeman MAR, Dean MRE, Hanham IWF. The etiology and prevention of functional instability of the foot. J Bone Joint Surg (B) 1965;47(4): 678–685.

[97] Mattiello-Rosa SM, Camargo PR, Santos AA. Abnormal isokinetic time-to-peak torque of the medial rotators of the shoulder in subjects with impingement syndrome. J Shoulder Elbow Surg 2008;17(1 Suppl): 54S–60S.

[98] Chapman AR, Vicenzino B, Blanch P, et al. Does cycling effect motor coordination of the leg during running in elite triathletes? J Sci Med Sport 2007;11(4):371–380[Epub 2007 Apr 26].

[99] Missitzi J, Geladas N, Klissouras V. Heritability in neuromuscular coordination: implications for motor control strategies. Med Sci Sports Exerc 2004;36(2):233–240.

[100] Alvares KM, Hulin CL. Two explanations of temporal changes in ability–skill relationship: a literature review and theoretical analysis. Hum Factors 1972;14:295–308.

[101] Fitts PM, Posner MI. Human performance. Pacific Grove, CA: Brooks/Cole; 1967.

[102] Airaksinen O, Herno A, Kaukanen E, et al. Density of lumbar muscles 4 years after decompressive spinal surgery. Eur Spine J 1996;5(3):193–197.

[103] Ng JK, Richardson CA, Kippers V, et al. Relationship between muscle fiber composition and functional capacity of back muscles in healthy subjects and patients

with back pain. J Orthop Sports Phys Ther 1998;27(6):389–402.

[104] Kristjansson E. Reliability of ultrasonography for the cervical multifidus muscle in asymptomatic and symptomatic subjects. Man Ther 2004; 9(2):83–88.

[105] Prushansky T. Cervical muscles weakness in chronic whiplash patients. Clin Biomech (Bristol, Avon) 2005;20(8):794–798.

[106] Andersen LL, Nielsen PK, Søgaard K. Torque–EMG–velocity relationship in female workers with chronic neck muscle pain. J Biomech 2008;41(9):2029–2035 [Epub 2008 May 5].

[107] Konishi Y, Ikeda K, Nishino A, et al. Relationship between quadriceps femoris muscle volume and muscle torque after anterior cruciate ligament repair. Scand J Med Sci Sports 2007; 17(6):656–661.

[108] Cools AM, Witvrouw EE, Mahieu NN, Danneels LA. Isokinetic scapular muscle performance in overhead athletes with and without impingement symptoms. J Athl Train 2005;40(2):104–110.

[109] Tyler TF, Nahow RC, Nicholas SJ, et al. Quantifying shoulder rotation weakness in patients with shoulder impingement. J Shoulder Elbow Surg 2005;14(6):570–574.

[110] Kamper DG, Harvey RL, Suresh S, et al. Relative contributions of neural mechanisms versus muscle mechanics in promoting finger extension deficits following stroke. Muscle Nerve 2003; 28(3):309–318.

[111] Kamper DG, Fischer HC, Cruz EG, et al. Weakness is the primary contributor to finger impairment in chronic stroke. Arch Phys Med Rehabil 2006; 87(9):1262–1269.

[112] Dall'Alba PT. Cervical range of motion discriminates between asymptomatic persons and those with whiplash. Spine 2001; 26(19):2090–2094.

[113] Vogt L, Segieth C, Banzer W, Himmelreich H. Movement behaviour in patients with

chronic neck pain. Physiother Res Int 2007;12(4):206–212.

[114] Berchuck M, Andriacchi TP. Gait adaptations by patients who have a deficient anterior cruciate ligament. J Bone Joint Surg Am 1990;72A:871–877.

[115] Hurd WJ, Snyder-Mackler L. Knee instability after acute ACL rupture affects movement patterns during the mid-stance phase of gait. J Orthop Res 2007;25(10):1369–1377.

[116] Thambyah A, Thiagarajan P, Goh Cho Hong J. Knee joint moments during stair climbing of patients with anterior cruciate ligament deficiency. Clin Biomech (Bristol, Avon) 2004;19(5):489–496.

[117] Mihaltchev P, Archambault PS, Feldman AG, et al. Control of double-joint arm posture in adults with unilateral brain damage. Exp Brain Res 2005;163(4):468–486.

[118] Beer RF, Dewald JP, Dawson ML, et al. Target-dependent differences between free and constrained arm movements in chronic hemiparesis. Exp Brain Res 2004;156(4):458–470.

[119] Sjölander P, Michaelson P, Jaric S, et al. Sensorimotor disturbances in chronic neck pain-range of motion, peak velocity, smoothness of movement, and repositioning acuity. Man Ther 2008; 13(2):122–131.

[120] Descarreaux M, Mayrand N, Raymond J. Neuromuscular control of the head in an isometric force reproduction task: comparison of whiplash subjects and healthy controls. Spine J 2007;7(6):647–653.

[121] Robon MJ, Perell KL, Fang M, et al. The relationship between ankle plantar flexor muscle moments and knee compressive forces in subjects with and without pain. Clin Biomech (Bristol, Avon) 2000; 15(7):522–527.

[122] Shrader MW, Draganich LF, Pottenger LA, et al. Effects of knee pain relief in osteoarthritis on gait and stair-stepping.

Clin Orthop Relat Res 2004; (421):188–193.

[123] Mündermann A, Dyrby CO, Hurwitz DE, et al. Potential strategies to reduce medial compartment loading in patients with knee osteoarthritis of varying severity: reduced walking speed. Arthritis Rheum 2004;50(4):1172–1178.

[124] Wirth B, van Hedel HJ, Curt A. Ankle dexterity is less impaired than muscle strength in incomplete spinal cord lesion. J Neurol 2008;255(2):273–279.

[125] Lamontagne A, Paquet N, Fung J. Postural adjustments to voluntary head motions during standing are modified following stroke. Clin Biomech (Bristol, Avon) 2003;18 (9):832–842.

[126] Mirbagheri MM, Tsao CC, Rymer WZ. Abnormal intrinsic and reflex stiffness related to impaired voluntary movement. Conf Proc IEEE Eng Med Biol Soc 2004;7:4680–4683.

[127] Lee H, Nicholson LL, Adams RD, et al. Proprioception and rotation range sensitization associated with subclinical neck pain. Spine 2005;30(3): E60–E67.

[128] Oksanen A, Pöyhönen T, Metsähonkala L, et al. Neck flexor muscle fatigue in adolescents with headache: an electromyographic study. Eur J Pain 2007;11(7):764–772.

[129] McHugh MP, Tyler TF, Nicholas SJ, et al. Electromyographic analysis of quadriceps fatigue after anterior cruciate ligament reconstruction. J Orthop Sports Phys Ther 2001;31(1):25–32.

[130] Snyder-Mackler L, Binder-Macleod SA, Williams PR. Fatigability of human quadriceps femoris muscle following anterior cruciate ligament reconstruction. Med Sci Sports Exerc 1993;25(7):783–789.

[131] van Lent ME, Drost MR, vd Wildenberg FA. EMG profiles of ACL-deficient patients during walking: the influence of mild fatigue. Int J Sports Med 1994;15(8):508–514.

[132] Sokk J, Gapeyeva H, Ereline J, et al. Shoulder muscle strength and fatigability in patients with frozen shoulder syndrome: the effect of 4-week individualized rehabilitation. Electromyogr Clin Neurophysiol 2007; 47(4–5):205–213.

[133] Nederhand MJ, Hermens HJ, IJzerman MJ, et al. Chronic neck pain disability due to an acute whiplash injury. Pain 2003;102(1–2):63–71.

[134] Fernández-de-Las-Peñas C, Falla D, Arendt-Nielsen L, Farina D. Cervical muscle co-activation in isometric contractions is enhanced in chronic tension-type headache patients. Cephalalgia 2008;28(7):744–751 [Epub 2008 May 5].

[135] Oksanen A, Pöyhönen T, Ylinen JJ. Force production and EMG activity of neck muscles in adolescent headache. Disabil Rehabil 2008;30(3):231–239.

[136] Torry MR, Decker MJ, Ellis HB, et al. Mechanisms of compensating for anterior cruciate ligament deficiency during gait. Med Sci Sports Exerc 2004;36(8):1403–1412.

[137] Ciccotti MG, Kerlan RK, Perry J, Pink M. An electromyographic analysis of the knee during functional activities. II. The anterior cruciate ligament-deficient and -reconstructed profiles. Am J Sports Med 1995;23:515–516.

[138] Kalund S, Sinkjaer T, Arendt-Nielsen L, Simonsen O. Altered timing of hamstring muscle action in anterior cruciate ligament deficient patients. Am J Sports Med 1990;18:245–248.

[139] Lass P, Kaalund S, leFevre S, et al. Muscle coordination following rupture of the anterior cruciate ligament: electromyographic studies of 14 patients. Acta Orthop Scand 1991;62:9–14.

[140] Chmielewski TL, Hurd WJ, Snyder-Mackler L. Elucidation of a potentially destabilizing control strategy in ACL deficient non-copers. J Electromyogr Kinesiol 2005; 15(1):83–92.

[141] Rudolph KS, Eastlack ME, Axe MJ, et al. Basmajian student award paper: Movement patterns after anterior cruciate ligament injury: a comparison of patients who compensate well for the injury and those who require operative stabilization. J Electromyogr Kinesiol 1998; 8(6):349–362.

[142] Lewek MD, Ramsey DK, Snyder-Mackler L. Knee stabilization in patients with medial compartment knee osteoarthritis. Arthritis Rheum 2005;52(9):2845–2853.

[143] Moraes GF, Faria CD, Teixeira-Salmela LF. Scapular muscle recruitment patterns and isokinetic strength ratios of the shoulder rotator muscles in individuals with and without impingement syndrome. J Shoulder Elbow Surg 2008;17 (Suppl. 1):48S–53S.

[144] Cools AM, Witvrouw EE, Declercq GA, et al. Scapular muscle recruitment patterns: trapezius muscle latency with and without impingement symptoms. Am J Sports Med 2003;31(4): 542–549.

[145] Kelly BT, Williams RJ, Cordasco FA. Differential patterns of muscle activation in patients with symptomatic and asymptomatic rotator cuff tears. J Shoulder Elbow Surg 2005; 14(2):165–171.

[146] Lin JJ, Wu YT, Wang SF, et al. Trapezius muscle imbalance in individuals suffering from frozen shoulder syndrome. Clin Rheumatol 2005;24(6): 569–575.

[147] Tedroff K, Knutson LM, Soderberg GL. Synergistic muscle activation during maximum voluntary contractions in children with and without spastic cerebral palsy. Dev Med Child Neurol 2006;48(10):789–796.

[148] Shum GL, Crosbie J, Lee RY. Symptomatic and asymptomatic movement coordination of the lumbar spine and hip during an everyday activity. Spine 2005; 30(23):E697–E702.

[149] Sjöström H, Allum JH, Carpenter MG, et al. Trunk

sway measures of postural stability during clinical balance tests in patients with chronic whiplash injury symptoms. Spine 2003;28(15):1725–1734.

[150] Eriksson PO, Zafar H, Häggman-Henrikson B. Deranged jaw-neck motor control in whiplash-associated disorders. Eur J Oral Sci 2004;112(1):25–32.

[151] Johnston V, Jull G, Darnell R, et al. Alterations in cervical muscle activity in functional and stressful tasks in female office workers with neck pain. Eur J Appl Physiol 2008;103(3):253–264 [Epub 2008 Feb 22].

[152] Johnston V, Jull G, Souvlis T, et al. Neck movement and muscle activity characteristics in female office workers with neck pain. Spine 2008;33(5): 555–563.

[153] Beer RF, Dewald JP, Rymer WZ. Deficits in the coordination of multijoint arm movements in patients with hemiparesis: evidence for disturbed control of limb dynamics. Exp Brain Res 2000;131(3):305–319.

[154] Musampa NK, Mathieu PA, Levin MF. Relationship between stretch reflex thresholds and voluntary arm muscle activation in patients with spasticity. Exp Brain Res 2007;181(4): 579–593.

[155] Lewis GN, Byblow WD. Bimanual coordination dynamics in poststroke hemiparetics. J Mot Behav 2004;36(2): 174–188.

[156] Ustinova KI, Fung J, Levin MF. Disruption of bilateral temporal coordination during arm swinging in patients with hemiparesis. Exp Brain Res 2006;169(2):194–207.

[157] McCombe Waller S, Whitall J. Fine motor control in adults with and without chronic hemiparesis: baseline comparison to nondisabled adults and effects of bilateral arm training. Arch Phys Med Rehabil 2004;85(7): 1076–1083.

[158] Popa T, Bonifazi M, della Volpe R, et al. Adaptive changes

in postural strategy selection in chronic low back pain. Exp Brain Res 2007;177(3):411–418.

[159] della Volpe R, Popa T, Ginanneschi F, et al. Changes in coordination of postural control during dynamic stance in chronic low back pain patients. Gait Posture 2006;24(3): 349–355.

[160] Bouche K, Stevens V, Cambier D, et al. Comparison of postural control in unilateral stance between healthy controls and lumbar discectomy patients with and without pain. Eur Spine J 2006;15(4):423–432.

[161] Mok NW, Brauer SG, Hodges PW. Hip strategy for balance control in quiet standing is reduced in people with low back pain. Spine 2004;29(6): E107–E112.

[162] Michaelson P, Michaelson M, Jaric S. Vertical posture and head stability in patients with chronic neck pain. J Rehabil Med 2003; 35(5):229–235.

[163] Giacomini PG, Alessandrini M, Evangelista M, et al. Impaired postural control in patients affected by tension-type headache. Eur J Pain 2004; 8(6):579–583.

[164] Luoto S, Taimela S, Hurri H, et al. Psychomotor speed and postural control in chronic low back pain patients. A controlled follow-up study. Spine 1996; 21(22):2621–2627.

[165] Wu CY, Chou SH, Chen CL, et al. Kinematic analysis of a functional and sequential bimanual task in patients with left hemiparesis: intra-limb and interlimb coordination. Disabil Rehabil 2008;26:1–9.

[166] Elert J, Kendall SA, Larsson B, et al. Chronic pain and difficulty in relaxing postural muscles in patients with fibromyalgia and chronic whiplash associated disorders. J Rheumatol 2001; 28(6):1361–1368.

[167] Larsson B, Björk J, Elert J, et al. Mechanical performance and electromyography during repeated maximal isokinetic

shoulder forward flexions in female cleaners with and without myalgia of the trapezius muscle and in healthy controls. Eur J Appl Physiol 2000; 83(4–5):257–267.

[168] Thorn S, Søgaard K, Kallenberg LA, et al. Trapezius muscle rest time during standardised computer work – a comparison of female computer users with and without self-reported neck/shoulder complaints. J Electromyogr Kinesiol 2007;17(4):420–427.

[169] Hurley MV, Newham DJ. The influence of arthrogenous muscle inhibition on quadriceps rehabilitation of patients with early, unilateral osteoarthritic knees. Br J Rheumatol 1993;32:127–131.

[170] Solomonow M, Baratta R, Zhou BH, et al. The synergistic action of the anterior cruciate ligament and thigh muscles in maintaining joint stability. Am J Sports Med 1987;15 (3):207–213.

[171] Ericsson YB, Dahlberg LE, Roos EM. Effects of functional exercise training on performance and muscle strength after meniscectomy: a randomized trial. Scand J Med Sci Sports 2008;19(2):156–165 [Epub 2008 Apr 6].

[172] Carpenter DM, Nelson BW. Low back strengthening for the prevention and treatment of low back pain. Med Sci Sports Exerc 1999;31(1):18–24.

[173] Danneels LA, Cools AM, Vanderstraeten GG, et al. The effects of three different training modalities on the cross-sectional area of the paravertebral muscles. Scand J Med Sci Sport 2001; 11(6):335–341.

[174] Kaser L, Mannion AF, Rhyner A, et al. Active therapy for chronic low back pain: part 2. Effects on paraspinal muscle cross-sectional area, fiber type size, and distribution. Spine 2001;26(8):909–919.

[175] Storheim K, Holm I, Gunderson R, et al. The effect of comprehensive group training on cross-sectional area, density, and strength of paraspinal muscles in patients sick-listed for subacute low back pain. J Spinal Disord Tech 2003; 16(3):271–279.

[176] Falla DL, Jull GA, Hodges PW. Patients with neck pain demonstrate reduced electromyographic activity of the deep cervical flexor muscles during performance of the craniocervical flexion test. Spine 2004;29(19):2108–2114.

[177] Ageberg E, Zatterstrom R, Moritz U, et al. Influence of supervised and nonsupervised training on postural control after an acute anterior cruciate ligament rupture: a three-year longitudinal prospective study. J Ortho Sports Phys Ther 2001;31(11):632–644.

[178] Eils E, Rosenbaum D. A multi-station proprioceptive exercise program in patients with ankle instability. Med Sci Sports Exerc 2001;33(12):1991–1998.

[179] Chmielewski TL, Hurd WJ, Rudolph KS, et al. Perturbation training improves knee kinematics and reduces muscle co-contraction after complete unilateral anterior cruciate ligament rupture. Phys Ther 2005;85(8):740–749 discussion 750–754.

[180] Hurd WJ, Chmielewski TL, Snyder-Mackler L. Perturbation-enhanced neuromuscular training alters muscle activity in female athletes. Knee Surg Sports Traumatol Arthrosc 2006;14(1):60–69.

[181] Wong AM, Lan C. Tai chi and balance control. Med Sport Sci 2008;52:115–123.

[182] Ihara H, Takayama M, Fukumoto T, 2008. Postural control capability of ACL-deficient knee after sudden tilting. Gait Posture May 9. [Epub ahead of print].

Sensory abilities

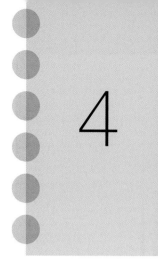

Sensory losses, and in particular proprioceptive deficits, may lead to unrefined movement and the loss of ability to respond effectively to sudden demands and may impede motor adaptation/learning. This chapter will examine how proprioceptive losses may come about and the underlying peripheral and central mechanisms seen in different conditions.

Sensory abilities include proprioception and exteroception (vision, vestibular apparatus and audition). Generally, clinical care of exteroception is out of the scope of neuromuscular rehabilitation. However, these sensory contributions should not be underestimated and their losses should be considered in the overall management of the patient.[1]

Sensory complexity model

Similar to motor abilities, sensory information can be categorized into groups of varying levels of complexity (Fig. 4.1).

Let us start with a simple movement such as elbow flexion–extension, preferably with the eyes shut. We can selectively focus our attention on the elbow before moving it. The awareness that the elbow is held at a particular angle is called *position sense*. As the elbow is moving, we now become aware of the direction, changes in velocity and acceleration–deceleration of the limb – a *movement sense*. There is also a *sense of effort* in moving and the limb's own weight (Ch. 2).[2,3,4] These elements of proprioception will be termed here as *primary proprioceptive ability*.

Now, let's make this a little more complex. With the eyes still shut, try to touch the tip of your nose with the index finger. Your ability (or inability) to accurately reach that target depends on the integration of sensory information from the whole arm, head and position of the nose; plus all the information from the rest of the body. This is *spatial orientation* ability: the capacity to identify the position and direction of movement of any part of the body.

Finally, imagine standing, balancing on one leg and then maintaining the same touch-the-nose movement. Your success depends on the capacity of the motor system to integrate several sources of exteroceptive (visual, vestibular and auditory) and proprioceptive information. This level of sensory ability will be termed here as *composite sensory ability*.

Hence, proprioception can be categorized according to complexity, from low to high level, as following:

- Primary proprioceptive ability (position, movement and effort sense)
- Spatial orientation
- Composite sensory ability.

It should be noted that this classification is artificial and that all these abilities co-exist in normal functional movement. However, this sensory ability model has some clinical value – it can be used as a predictive tool to understand potential sensory losses in relation to various conditions. It can also provide a useful clinical procedure for testing more obvious losses and integrating sensory with motor rehabilitation. The assessment and challenges of proprioception are described in Chapter 13.

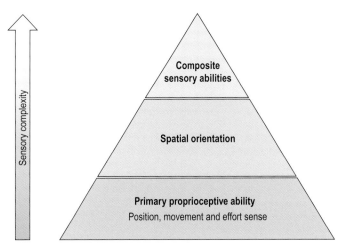

Fig. 4.1 • Sensory complexity model. Principal sensory abilities are position, movement and effort sense. Next in complexity is the integration of proprioception from several sources to provide a sense of the position and movement of the whole limb in space. The integration of visual, auditory, vestibular and proprioceptive is represented as composite sensory ability.

Change in proprioceptive acuity

Proprioceptive acuity refers to a change in the ability of the individual to detect various aspects of movement. It can be the threshold to rate and amplitude of movement; for example, if the movement is very slow the individual may find it hard to identify whether the limb is moving at all and in which direction.[5] Acuity is also the ability to detect a joint's angle when maintained in a certain position or dynamically during movement.

Proprioceptive acuity depends on the intactness of the sensing apparatus (mechanoreceptors and their peripheral to central pathways) and the intactness of central integration/possessing of sensory information.[6] Generally, in musculoskeletal injury the damage is to the proprioceptive apparatus in the periphery. Later it may be accompanied by adaptive central reorganization. Conversely, in central nervous system (CNS) damage, the peripheral proprioceptive apparatus is fully intact but the centres that process the information are damaged.

Proprioceptive changes in musculoskeletal injury

Proprioceptive changes in musculoskeletal injuries often manifest as diminished acuity in position and movement sense.[7-10] These changes together with

nociception often result in unrefined motor control (Fig. 4.2). Proprioceptive deficits have been demonstrated in the ankle,[11] knee,[12-15] shoulder,[16] temporomandibular joint,[8] lower back,[17-20] and neck (whiplash injuries).[21-23] Chronic neck pain was even shown to reduce acuity in upper limb (elbow, shoulder and spatial orientation of whole arm), suggesting a central processing change in sensory integration.[24-26]

Various degrees of musculoskeletal injuries, surgical intervention and degenerative joint disease have been shown to have local effects on proprioception.[27-34]

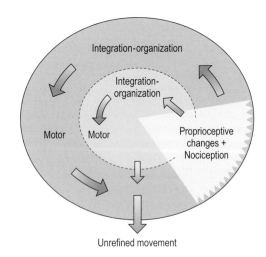

Fig. 4.2 • Damage to proprioceptive apparatus peripherally combined with nociception will result in unrefined motor output.

The clinical significance of proprioceptive losses is not clear. For example in severe neck pain conditions the losses are often less than 2.5° of error when compared to asymptomatic subjects.[20,35,36] With more mild conditions, often the differences between symptomatic and asymptomatic subjects are less that 1° in proprioceptive error.[22,37–41] It should be noted that even asymptomatic individuals can demonstrate up to 5° in proprioceptive error.[38,41]

Short-term, reversible proprioceptive changes

There is a common experience that following intense exercise we tend to feel unsteady (wobbly legs) and clumsy in the execution of skilled movements. This unrefined movement may be partly associated with the exercise-induced muscle damage and the effects it has on proprioception. Such proprioceptive changes are self-limiting and are expected to recover within minutes in the case of fatigue, or longer in the case of delayed muscle soreness after exercise.[10,42–48]

The changes in proprioception are generally modest. For example, immediately after eccentric quadriceps exercise there is a force drop of 28%, accompanied by 4.8 degrees of error. Following concentric exercise, there is a force drop of 15% and matching errors of 3.7 degrees.[43] On the other hand, proprioceptive acuity may increase during normal warm-up where there is no fatigue or muscle damage.[49]

Several factors may contribute to this transient change in proprioception. Muscle swelling and sarcomere damage may influence the ability of the muscle receptors to effectively detect movement (Fig. 4.3). Furthermore, ischaemia or inflammation is known to change the chemical environment of

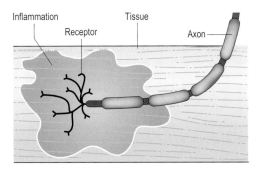

Fig. 4.3 • Changes in the chemical environment of the mechanoreceptor may change its sensitivity in detecting movement.

the muscle receptors and their sensitivity (group III and IV chemosensitive afferents and the spindle afferents via spinal mechanisms).[50–54]

There may be also central reasons for transient changes in acuity. During eccentric exercise the efferent motor command may increase to compensate for the effects of fatigue. The proprioceptive errors are due to inaccurate comparison between predicted and actual feedback from the muscle (see comparator system, Ch. 2).[43]

Generally, these acute transient changes in proprioceptive acuity have little clinical implications and are unlikely to be affected by any special rehabilitative approach. In long-term injury or ongoing painful conditions they may become more permanent and, therefore, more relevant to rehabilitation (see below).

Where transient proprioception may be important is in sports management, particularly in the area of injury prevention during training and competition. During fatigue skillful movement may deteriorate, due to a combination of several factors, including reduced proprioceptive acuity (also reduced motor control and psychological-cognitive factors).[55–57] These multidimensional factors may place the athlete in movement patterns that could predispose them to injury.[58–61] The management of the athlete in this situation would involve the organization-behaviour of the individual, which is further discussed in Chapter 8.

Long-term proprioceptive changes

Long-term reversible and irreversible proprioceptive changes can be observed in musculoskeletal injuries. Several factors can combine to generate these changes:

* Damage to the receptors and/or their axons
* Structural-physical changes of the tissue in which the receptor is embedded
* Central sensory reorganization
* Pain-proprioception competition.

Many receptors and their axons have a lower tensile strength compared to the tissues in which they are embedded. Physical trauma to tissues and nerve trunks can damage the mechanoreceptors and their axons resulting in localized proprioceptive losses (Fig.4.4A).[14,15,31,61–64] These proprioceptive deficits can be very small and their clinical significance is unknown. For example, in cruciate ligament tears it can be less then 1.0 degree of movement.[65]

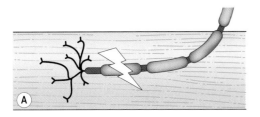

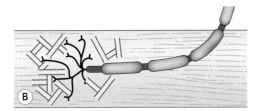

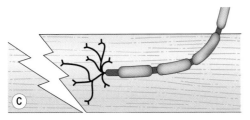

Fig. 4.4 • Local changes affecting the proprioceptive apparatus. **A**, Damage to the receptor or its axon. **B**, Changes in the tissues in which the receptor is embedded. **C**, Torn fibres will reduce the receptor's ability to detect mechanical changes.

Another potential mechanism that may lead to long-term sensory losses is structural/physical change in the tissues in which the receptor is embedded. The proprioceptive apparatus may be fully intact, but its ability to detect movement may be hindered by changes in the surrounding tissues, in the form of adhesions or shortening (Fig. 4.4B). Furthermore, proprioceptors embedded in tissues that are torn or detached will lack the mechanical stimulation needed for the detection of movement (Fig. 4.4C).

Central sensory reorganization in response to injury may also influence long-term changes in proprioception. Reduced physical activity may result in sensory "disuse", affecting the whole sensory continuum from the receptors to their central representation in the brain. For example, in the periphery, immobilization can lead to muscle spindle atrophy and changes in its sensitivity and firing rate.[66] More centrally, it has been shown that tactile impoverishment and sensorimotor restriction of an animal's paw causes deterioration in the cortical sensory map representing that area.[67]

The reversal of disuse may be observed after reconstructive capsular and ligamentous surgery. Once repaired, proprioception tends to recover over a period of several months.[68–71] This partly could be due to the patient's returning to a more normal and pain-free use of the arm that promotes normal central reorganization of proprioception.[73]

Central sensory reorganization can produce surprising findings. In individuals who had anterior cruciate ligament (ACL) reconstruction or shoulder injury, decreased proprioceptive ability was present in some measurements in the affected, as well as in the uninjured side.[73–77]

Competition in sensory information: nociception vs. proprioception?

Changes in proprioceptive acuity after injury could be due to a competition between nociception and proprioception for central "attention," occurring at reflexive and cognitive levels.[50,51,53,77]

This competition in sensory information can be likened to a bottleneck effect. A vast array of information from the periphery floods the CNS. The system is incapable of attending to all these inputs and, therefore, only information which is relevant or important makes it through to attention. Pain, which may be interpreted as being the most important, will have dominance over proprioception in passing through this bottleneck of information.

There are several studies which support this sensory competition model. Experimental pain induced in muscle and subcutaneous tissues was shown to significantly impair passive movement detection in the pertaining joint.[79] Proprioceptive acuity has been shown to reduce when experimental pain was induced in the muscles of the lower leg[80] and, likewise, superficial experimental pain applied locally to the neck diminished neck proprioceptive acuity.[81] Such sensory competition was also demonstrated in postural stability. When a painful heat stimulus was applied to the skin of the calf it resulted in greater postural unsteadiness.[82]

Pain-proprioception competition is also evident in musculoskeletal injury. Patients with painful ACL damage seem to have larger proprioceptive deficits than those who have pain-free ACL damage.[83] It was also demonstrated that proprioception improves after 6 months following shoulder decompression surgery where only the inflamed and painful subaccromial bursa was removed, i.e. proprioception won when the competition (pain) was taken out.[71]

Another possibility for pain-proprioception competition may occur, more centrally, as an adaptive process. This phenomenon may be related to the principle that the more we focus on an experience such as a physical sensation or movement, the more it drives central adaptation.[84-88] In this scenario the individual's focus on their pain may facilitate pain imprinting while displacing normal sensory-motor central representation. For example, in chronic lower back pain there is a displacement of the cortical sensory-motor areas representing the lower back[89] and, indeed, this condition is often accompanied by diminished proprioceptive acuity.[16-19]

Proprioceptive changes in central nervous system damage

CNS damage could also lead to sensory losses. Depending on the extent and location of damage, all levels of sensory abilities may be affected. This is in contrast to musculoskeletal injuries where the primary proprioceptive abilities are largely affected. Another important difference is that in CNS damage the peripheral sensory apparatus is left intact, which provides a potential for peripheral-to-central recovery (Fig. 4.5). This however depends on the extent of the damage, neural repair and central reorganization (Ch. 10).[90-94]

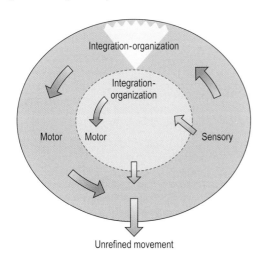

Fig. 4.5 • Central damage can affect proprioception. In contrast to musculoskeletal injuries the proprioceptive apparatus remains still intact.

Proprioceptive recovery

Proprioceptive losses will partially or fully recover during a period of several months following musculoskeletal injury. The recovery of proprioception ultimately relies on peripheral and central processes: in the periphery, through the degree of repair of the receptors and the tissue in which they are embedded, and centrally, through the adaptation and reorganization of the sensory pathways and cortical maps.

There is some evidence that mechanoreceptors can partially regenerate following tissue damage. Such regeneration has been shown in muscle spindles, their axons and efferent motor supply and in skin mechanoreceptors (Fig. 4.6).[63,64,95-97] In animal models there has been even some evidence for sprouting of new muscle and skin receptors, which took place within 6 weeks of injury.[64,97,98] In muscle, the success of regeneration depends on the extent of internal damage and scarring and the duration of repair.

Being active is important for sensory regeneration. Muscle hypertrophy in response to exercising is associated with morphological and physiological changes of the muscle spindle. Such changes will increase the spindle's sensitivity to detect movement.[99-101] Centrally, exercise encourages the sensory neurons to produce growth factors that stimulate axonal regeneration and synaptic connections (Fig. 4.7).[102]

The recovery of the tissue in which the receptors are embedded is also important for proprioception.[103] Naturally occurring healing or surgical repair could lead to normalization of the tissue's properties and consequently to better detection of movement by the receptors embedded in them. Some evidence of such recovery was demonstrated following spinal, ankle and shoulder surgery.[68-72,104] It is possible that in some of these surgical repairs the tensions in the capsule had been restored, consequently re-establishing the receptors' detection ability in the previously torn fibres (this does not occur in every surgical intervention, e.g. cruciate ligament).[74] This suggests that passive or active movement may be advantageous for such sensory regeneration. It will optimize tissue repair, reduce oedema and scarring as well as optimize the mechanical environment necessary for receptor regeneration/adaptation.[105]

The feedback from the spared receptors in the area of damage as well as from receptors from undamaged areas could also account for the recovery of proprioception (rather than through an

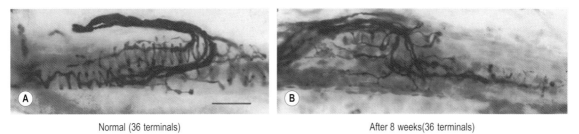

Normal (36 terminals)   After 8 weeks(36 terminals)

Fig. 4.6 • Muscle spindle regeneration after damage to the nerve trunk. **A,** Normal spindle afferents (36 terminals). **B,** Regeneration after 8 weeks (36 terminals). (From Barker D, Scott JJ 1990 Regeneration and recovery of cat muscle spindles after devascularization. J Physiol 424:27–39, with permission).

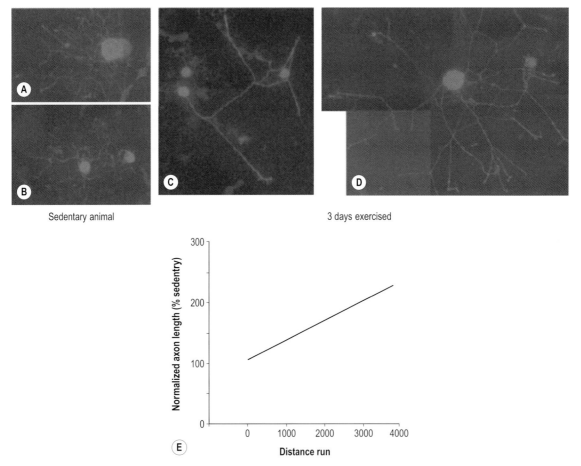

Fig. 4.7 • Exercise encourages the release of growth factors by sensory neurons that stimulate axonal regeneration and formation of new synaptic connections. A and B, Sedentary animal. C and D, Three days exercised. E correlation between distance run and normalized axon length (From Molteni R, Zheng JQ, Ying Z et al 2004 Voluntary exercise increases axonal regeneration from sensory neurons. Proc Natl Acad Sci USA 101(22):8473–8478 (Fig. 1), with permission.)

improvement of proprioception from the area of damage itself).[106,107] In this scenario, the spared proprioceptors become more dominant and capture the lost central representation of the damaged receptors (Fig. 4.8). Such loss and recapture of somatosensory cortical territory has been observed during denervation and re-innervation of peripheral nerve and in the proximal limbs of amputees (Ch. 6).[108] The other possibility is that the receptors that were damaged gradually regain their lost

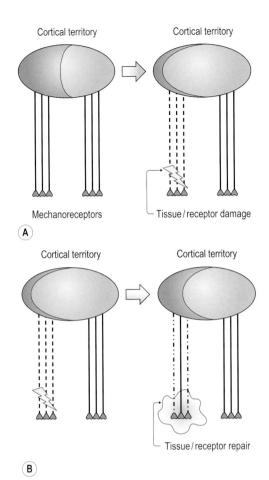

Cortical territory   Cortical territory

Mechanoreceptors   Tissue/receptor damage

A

Cortical territory   Cortical territory

Tissue/receptor repair

B

Fig. 4.8 • Mechanisms in proprioceptive recovery.
A, Damage to the receptors or the tissue in which they are embedded could lead to loss in their cortical representation and capture of that area by the saved receptors. Some proprioceptive recovery may be possible by the system becoming more dependent on the saved receptors and their enlarged cortical representation; even if there is no further recovery of the damaged receptor or tissue. B, Gradual repair of the receptor or the tissue in which it is embedded may help recapture its lost cortical representation and improve overall proprioception from the area of injury.

central territory as they regenerate and become more functional. Here too we can assume that active movement is the drive to sensory-motor plasticity. This was demonstrated in stroke patients. Functional rehabilitation brought about improvement in motor control that correlates with reorganization in the somatosensory cortex.[109]

In can be concluded that after musculoskeletal injuries or CNS damage there is a potential for proprioceptive recovery. The studies suggest that recovery is a mix of repair and adaptation processes that occur

throughout the sensory system.[110] As such, proprioceptive recovery is expected to take several months rather than a few weeks. Often such intrinsic body processes can be optimized but not speeded up. Movement may help this optimization by facilitating tissue repair and providing the drive for central sensory-motor adaptation.[110] However, the degree and time-scale of recovery may be difficult to predetermine.[111]

Clinical note

• Movement can help optimize repair and adaption of the proprioceptive system.
• Movement will also help the repair and adaption of the tissues in which the receptors are embedded. This may help to re-establish the receptors' ability to detect movement.

Does proprioceptive loss lead to further damage?

Proprioceptive loss in the long-term *is believed* to contribute to muscular atrophy, recurrent joint injuries and eventually to progressive degenerative joint disease.[46] In this model, diminished feedback will result in dysfunctional movement and joint instability, which will eventually lead to progressive joint damage. So far this model has been demonstrated only in one animal study.[112]

Functional instability of the ankle is a condition which can be used to examine this theory. It is well established that a combination of sensory-motor losses at the ankle may predispose the individual to recurrent injury.[11] Will this recurrent injury predispose the individual to progressive ankle joint damage? In a 20-year follow-up study of patients with chronic ankle instability, degenerative changes were observed only in six of 46 ankles. There was no correlation between persistent instability and joint degeneration.[113]

Another area that could help us to explore the proprioceptive further damage model is delayed-onset muscle soreness (DOMS) after exercise. This transient muscle condition is accompanied by diminished proprioceptive acuity.[10,42–48] Most individuals who experience DOMS will continue to exercise without acquiring any further damage/injury. If proprioceptive loss were to lead to injury, continuing to exercise would initiate a vicious cycle that would result in progressive damage.

Finally, in a recent prospective cohort study with 2–3 year follow-up the lumbar spine position sense was evaluated in 292 athletes. No significant differences in the repositioning errors or motion perception threshold between athletes with and without a history of lower back injury or between those who did and did not get injured during the follow-up.[135]

Clinical note

There is no evidence yet that proprioceptive losses predispose the individual to gradual tissue damage. Perhaps large magnitude proprioceptive losses are required for this chain of events to occur.

Are there proprioceptive-specific exercises?

Patients who exhibit proprioceptive losses are often prescribed specific proprioceptive exercise. Is there a distinct kind of exercise and would it be better than any other functional activity?

Let's take a look at the body – our ankle mechanoreceptors will be stimulated equally well whether we exercise on a wobble board or jump around the court while playing tennis. Indeed, the improvements in function or reported reduced incidents of injury after proprioceptive training are often attributed to enhancing motor control (e.g. synergistic control or coordination) rather than selective improvements in proprioception.[74,76,106,107,114–117]

Yet, some studies do show that in musculoskeletal injuries there are some direct and local improvements in position sense following "proprioception training"[118–120] However, it seems that proprioception improves regardless of the type of exercise used. For example, proprioceptive acuity in the shoulder seems to improve with isokinetic exercises, lifting weights, exercises which mimic the movement of lifting weights, push-ups, arm movement using a resistance band or throwing a weighted ball.[121–124]

If you feel baffled by all these findings, you should. How can specific exercises improve proprioception while the normal daily or sports activities of the individual do not? It could be that we become more attentive to proprioception rather than improving it. Imagine a simple task like writing. Once learned it becomes completely autonomous and out of our awareness. The focus of writing is external towards the goals of writing. If we were to increase the duration of writing the awareness and proprioception acuity of the hand will remain unchanged. So doing more of the same is unlikely to change proprioception. Now imagine that we were given a novel task that forced us to concentrate on our hand, say knitting. We have to become more aware of the fine hand movements of this new complex task. If we were to test proprioception of the hand at that point we may find that acuity has increased. This has come about because we are more attentive and focused on our hands, rather than by an improvement in proprioception. An analogy can be experienced by focusing to listening with your right ear. You will become more aware of the sound on that side; however, your hearing has not improved. Interestingly, it is claimed that elderly Tai chi practitioners have better proprioceptive acuity than their age-matched runners or swimmers and those who are non and exercising.[125,126] Is it because Tai chi uses more focus and attention on the body (see Internal and external focus and learning, Ch. 5)?

Another possible mechanism for increased acuity may be related to the comparator system. When a new activity is introduced the comparator system becomes more engaged in error detection. The sense of effort, which is a part of this system, may consequently become more co-active. It could be that the increases in the sense of effort will temporarily enhance proprioceptive acuity.

The short of it is that as long as the individual is doing a novel exercise, awareness of proprioception may increase and give the false impression that the proprioception is improving. It would be interesting to see what would happen to proprioceptive acuity after several months when that exercise is no longer novel, and is autonomous and boring.

Clinical note

- There is no specific proprioceptive exercise. All activities are likely to be equally effective.

Proprioception and prevention of injury

There is a commonly held belief that proprioceptive exercise or training can improve proprioceptive acuity and, therefore, prevent sports-related injuries.[127] The exercises that are prescribed often aim to challenge postural stability; they are performed at higher speeds and involve sudden unexpected perturbations, such as exercising on a wobble board (ankle disc exercise).[117]

In sports, most injuries occur during very rapid movements. Under such conditions the foot–ground impact force takes less than 50 ms to reach its peak magnitude and ankle inversion can reach 17° in as little as 40 ms. The swiftness of these events does not leave sufficient time for even the shortest spinal reflexes to execute an adequate motor response to prevent injury.[128] This lag in proprioceptive transmission time is immutable; it cannot be shortened by exercising. From a proprioceptive perspective, exercise cannot offer protection against injuries that occur during movement at medium to high velocities.

Furthermore, proprioceptive exercises on a wobble board are relatively slow, in the range of several hundreds of milliseconds. They are, therefore, unlikely to provide an optimal sensory training to protect the ankle against injury; even at medium movement velocities.[128] (A Cochrane systematic review suggests only limited evidence for the efficacy of wobble board use for prevention of ankle injury.)[129]

Proprioceptive acuity and passive and active movement

Are passive manual techniques useful for rehabilitation of proprioceptive or motor control? Proprioceptive acuity tends to increase when the

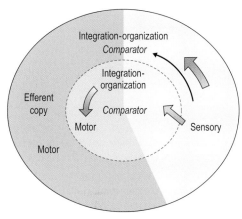

Fig. 4.10 • Passive movement engages only the sensory element within the motor process. It will fail to activate the comparator system. This will reduce the potential for learning movement, modifying it as well as excluding the sense of effort.

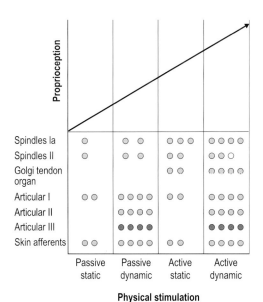

Fig. 4.9 • Proprioceptive acuity tends to rise when the physical stimulation is more dynamic and active (circles denotes excitation of receptor).

movement is more dynamic and active rather than passive (Fig. 4.9).[130,131] When a subject's joint is moved passively, the ability to distinguish the finger's position is reduced compared to when the subject slightly stiffens their finger during the movement.[2,132,133] This is reflected in more extensive cortical activity during active, in comparison to passive, movement.[134] It has also been proposed that the superiority of position sense in active motion is related to the efferent flow and the sense of effort (Ch. 2).[130] In active movement feedback is derived from both proprioception and this internal feedback, whereas passive motion tend to only stimulate the feedback portion of the motor system (Fig. 4.10).

This difference between active and passive motion was demonstrated in a recent study. Continuous active motion was compared with continuous passive motion for recovery of proprioception immediately after ACL reconstruction (unfortunately no control).[135] Significantly better results were obtained in the active motion group (4.2 ± 1.6 vs. 1.9 ± 1.2 degrees).

Summary points

- The sensory-motor system is a functional unit. There is no need to specifically target proprioception.
- Proprioceptive ability can be classified according to complexity from primary proprioceptive ability, spatial orientation ability to composite sensory ability.

49

- Proprioceptive acuity can be affected by peripheral and/or central causes.
- Musculoskeletal injury can affect the peripheral proprioceptive apparatus while CNS damage will affect central processing of proprioception.
- Recovery of proprioception involves both reparative and adaptive processes. As such, it may have its own inherent recovery period that may take several weeks or months to complete.
- Promoting normal functional movement will help proprioception by facilitating positive sensory-motor reorganization/adaptation.

- Recovery of proprioception is important for optimising movement control. It is still unclear if it provides protective function against future damage.
- There is no evidence that proprioceptive losses will result in long-term degenerative changes.
- Many of the proprioceptive changes seen after musculoskeletal injuries are very small and may have little or no impact on a person's functionality. It seems that the body can tolerate such minor changes.
- All exercises are proprioceptive exercises.
- Active movement is better than passive movement in stimulating proprioception.
- Message to the patient – "keep on moving".

References

[1] Treleaven J, LowChoy N, Darnell R, et al. Comparison of sensorimotor disturbance between subjects with persistent whiplash-associated disorder and subjects with vestibular pathology associated with acoustic neuroma. Arch Phys Med Rehabil 2008; 89(3):522–530.

[2] Gandevia SC, Smith JL, Crawford M, et al. Motor commands contribute to human position sense. J Physiol 2006; 571(Pt 3):703–710.

[3] Gill KP, Callaghan MJ. The measurement of lumbar proprioception in individuals with and without low back pain. Spine 1998;23(3):371–377.

[4] Gandevia SC, McCloskey DI, Burke D. Kinaesthetic signals and muscle contraction. Trends Neurosci 1992;15(2):64–65.

[5] Taylor JL, McCloskey DI. Detection of movement imposed at the elbow during active flexion in man. J Physiol 1992;457:503–513.

[6] Bard C, Paillard J, Lajoie Y, et al. Role of afferent information in the timing of motor commands: a comparative study with a deafferented patient. Neuropsychologia 1992; 30(2):201–206.

[7] Izacsson G, Isberg A, Persson A. Loss of directional orientation control of lower jaw movements in persons with internal derangement of the temporomandibular joint. Oral Surg 1988;66(1):8–12.

[8] Miall RC, Ingram HA, Cole JD, Gauthier GM. Weight estimation in a "deafferented" man and in control subjects: are judgements influenced by peripheral or central signals? Exp Brain Res 2000;133(4):491–500.

[9] Saxton JM, Clarkson PM, James R, et al. Neuromuscular dysfunction following eccentric exercise. Med Sci Sports Exerc 1995;27(8):1185–1193.

[10] Freeman MAR, Dean MRE, Hanham IWF. The etiology and prevention of functional instability of the foot. J Bone Joint Surg (B) 1965;47(4): 678–685.

[11] Barrack RL, Skinner HB, Cook SD, et al. Effect of articular disease and total knee arthroplasty on knee joint-position sense. J Neurophysiol 1983;50(3):684–687.

[12] Barrack RL, Skinner HB, Buckley SL. Proprioception in the anterior cruciate deficient knee. Am J Sports Med 1989;17(1): 1–6.

[13] Bonfim TR, Jansen Paccola CA, Barela JA. Proprioceptive and behavior impairments in individuals with anterior cruciate ligament reconstructed knees. Arch Phys Med Rehabil 2003;84:1217–1223.

[14] Fischer-Rasmussen T, Jensen PE. Proprioceptive sensitivity and performance in anterior cruciate ligament-deficient knee joints. Scand J Med Sci Sports 2000; 10(2):85–89.

[15] Myers JB, Lephart SM. Sensorimotor deficits contributing to glenohumeral instability. Clin Orthop 2002;400:98–104.

[16] Brumagne S, Cordo P, Lysens R, et al. The role of paraspinal muscle spindles in lumbosacral position sense in individuals with and without low back pain. Spine 2000;25(8):989–994.

[17] Givoni NJ, Pham T, Allen TJ, Proske U. The effect of quadriceps muscle fatigue on position matching at the knee. J Physiol 2007;584(Pt 1): 111–119.

[18] O'Sullivan PB, Burnett A, Floyd AN, et al. Lumbar repositioning deficit in a specific low back pain population. Spine 2003;28(10):1074–1079.

[19] Parkhurst TM, Burnett CN. Injury and proprioception in the lower back. J Orthop Sports Phys Ther 1994;19(5):282–295.

[20] Feipel V, Salvia P, Klein H. Head repositioning accuracy in patients with whiplash-associated disorders. Spine 2006;31(2): E51–E58.

[21] Loudon JK, Ruhl M, Field E. Ability to reproduce head position after whiplash injury. Spine 1997;22(8):865–868.

[22] Treleaven J, Jull G, LowChoy N. The relationship of cervical joint

position error to balance and eye movement disturbances in persistent whiplash. Man Ther 2006;11:99–106.

[23] Knox JJ, Beilstein DJ, Charles SD, et al. Changes in head and neck position have a greater effect on elbow joint position sense in people with whiplash-associated disorders. Clin J Pain 2006;22(6): 512–518.

[24] Sandlund J, Djupsjöbacka M, Ryhed B, et al. Predictive and discriminative value of shoulder proprioception tests for patients with whiplash-associated disorders. J Rehabil Med 2006; 38(1):44–49.

[25] Sandlund J, Röijezon U, Björklund M. Acuity of goal-directed arm movements to visible targets in chronic neck pain. J Rehabil Med 2008;40(5): 366–374.

[26] Barrett DS, Cobb AG, Bentley G. Joint proprioception in normal, osteoarthritic and replaced knee. J Bone Joint Surg (B) 1991; 73(1):53–56.

[27] Hassan BS, Mockett S, Doherty M. Static postural sway, proprioception, and maximal voluntary quadriceps contraction in patients with knee osteoarthritis and normal control subjects. Ann Rheum Dis 2001;60(6):612–618.

[28] Hurley MV, Scott DL, Rees J, et al. Sensorimotor changes and functional performance in patients with knee osteoarthritis. Ann Rheum Dis 1997;56(11): 641–648.

[29] Hurley MV, Rees J, Newham DJ. Quadriceps function, proprioceptive acuity and functional performance in healthy young, middle-aged and elderly subjects. Age Ageing 1998;27(1): 55–62.

[30] Safran MR, Allen AA, Lephart SM, et al. Proprioception in the posterior cruciate ligament deficient knee. Knee Surg Sports Traumatol Arthrosc 1999;7(5): 310–317.

[31] Sharma L. Proprioceptive impairment in knee osteoarthritis. Rheum Dis Clin N Am 1999; 25(2):299–314.

[32] Stauffer RN, Chao EYS, Gyory AN. Biomechanical gait analysis of the diseased knee joint. Clin Orthop 1977;126:246–255.

[33] Thomas PA, Andriacchhi TP, Galante JO, et al. Influence of total knee replacement design on walking and stair climbing. J Bone Joint Surg (A) 1982;64(9): 1328–1335.

[34] Heikkilä HV, Wenngren BI. Cervicocephalic kinesthetic sensibility, active range of cervical motion, and oculomotor function in patients with whiplash injury. Arch Phys Med Rehabil 1998; 79(9):1089–1094.

[35] Sjölander P, Michaelson P, Jaric S, et al. Sensorimotor disturbances in chronic neck pain–range of motion, peak velocity, smoothness of movement, and repositioning acuity. Man Ther 2008; 13(2):122–1231.

[36] Armstrong BS, McNair PJ, Williams M. Head and neck position sense in whiplash patients and healthy individuals and the effect of the cranio-cervical flexion action. Clin Biomech (Bristol, Avon) 2005; 20(7):675–684.

[37] Armstrong B, McNair P, Taylor D. Head and neck position sense. Sports Med 2008;38(2): 101–117.

[38] Friden T, Roberts D, Zatterstrom R, et al. Proprioception after an acute knee ligament injury: a longitudinal study on 16 consecutive patients. J Orthop Res 1997;15(5):637–644.

[39] Sterling M, Jull G, Vicenzino B, et al. Development of motor system dysfunction following whiplash injury. Pain 2003; 103(1–2):65–73.

[40] Teng CC, Chai H, Lai DM, et al. Cervicocephalic kinesthetic sensibility in young and middle-aged adults with or without a history of mild neck pain. Man Ther 2007;12(1):22–28.

[41] Carpenter JE, Blasier RB, Pellizzon GG. The effects of muscle fatigue on shoulder joint position sense. Am J Sports Med 1998;26(2):262–265.

[42] Glencross D, Thornton E. Position sense following injury. J Sports Med 1981;21:23–27.

[43] Hiemstra LA, Lo IK, Fowler PJ. Effect of fatigue on knee proprioception: implications for dynamic stabilization. J Orthop Sports Phys Ther 2001;31(10): 598–605.

[44] Marks R. Effects of exercise-induced fatigue on position sense of the knee. Aust J Physiother 1994;40(3):175–181.

[45] Skinner HB, Barrack RL, Cook SD, et al. Joint position sense in total knee arthroplasty. J Orthop Res 1984;1:276–283.

[46] Taimela S, Kankaanpaa M, Luoto S. The effect of lumbar fatigue on the ability to sense a change in lumbar position. A controlled study. Spine 1999;24(13):1322–1327.

[47] Tripp BL, Yochem EM, Uhl TL. Recovery of upper extremity sensorimotor system acuity in baseball athletes after a throwing-fatigue protocol. J Athl Train 2007;42(4):452–457.

[48] Bartlett MJ, Warren PJ. Effect of warming up on knee proprioception before sporting activity. Br J Sports Med 2002; 36(2):132–134.

[49] Johansson H, Djupsjobacka M, Sjolander P. Influence on the gamma-muscle spindle system from muscle afferents stimulated by KCl and lactic acid. Neurosci Res 1993;16(1):49–57.

[50] Martin PG, Weerakkody N, Gandevia SC, Taylor JL. Group III and IV muscle afferents differentially affect the motor cortex and motoneurones in humans. J Physiol 2008; 586(5):1277–1289.

[51] Pedersen J, Sjölander P, Wenngren BI, Johansson H. Increased intramuscular concentration of bradykinin increases the static fusimotor drive to muscle spindles in neck muscles of the cat. Pain 1997;70(1):83–91.

[52] Pedersen J, Ljubizavljevic M, Bergenheim M, et al. Alterations in information transmission in ensembles of primary muscle spindle afferents after muscle fatigue in heteronymous muscle.

Neuroscience 1998;84 (3):953–959.

[53] Thunberg J, Ljubizavljevic M, Djupsjöbacka M, Johansson H. Effects on the fusimotor-muscle spindle system induced by intramuscular injections of hypertonic saline. Exp Brain Res 2002;142(3):319–326.

[54] Cresswell SL, Eklund RC. Changes in athlete burnout over a thirty-week "rugby year" J Sci Med Sport 2006;9(1–2): 125–134.

[55] Orishimo KF, Kremenic IJ. Effect of fatigue on single-leg hop landing biomechanics. J Appl Biomech 2006;22(4):245–254.

[56] Murian A, Deschamps T, Bourbousson J, et al. Influence of an exhausting muscle exercise on bimanual coordination stability and attentional demands. Neurosci Lett 2008;432 (1):64–68.

[57] Borotikar BS, Newcomer R, Koppes R, et al. Combined effects of fatigue and decision making on female lower limb landing postures: central and peripheral contributions to ACL injury risk. Clin Biomech (Bristol, Avon) 2008;23(1):81–92.

[58] Chappell JD, Herman DC, Knight BS, et al. Effect of fatigue on knee kinetics and kinematics in stop-jump tasks. Am J Sports Med 2005;33(7):1022–1029.

[59] Kernozek TW, Torry MR, Iwasaki M. Gender differences in lower extremity landing mechanics caused by neuromuscular fatigue. Am J Sports Med 2008;36(3):554–565.

[60] McLean SG, Felin RE, Suedekum N, et al. Impact of fatigue on gender-based high-risk landing strategies. Med Sci Sports Exerc 2007;39(3):502–514.

[61] Barrack RL. Proprioception and function after anterior cruciate reconstruction. J Bone Joint Surg (B) 1991;73:833–837.

[62] Barker D, Scott JJ, Stacey MJ. Reinnervation and recovery of cat muscle receptors after long-term denervation. Exp Neurol 1986;94(1):184–202.

[63] Kolosova LI, Nozdrachev AD, Moiseeva AB, et al. Recovery of mechanoreception at the initial stage of regeneration of injured sciatic nerve in rats in conditions of central axotomy of sensory neurons. Neurosci Behav Physiol 2004;34(8):817–820.

[64] Beynnon BD, Good L, Risberg MA. The effect of bracing on proprioception of knees with anterior cruciate ligament injury. J Orthop Sports Phys Ther 2002;32(1):11–15.

[65] Maier A, Eldred E, Edgerton VR. The effect on spindles of muscle atrophy and hypertrophy. Exp Neurol 1972;37:100–123.

[66] Coq JO, Xerri C. Tactile impoverishment and sensorimotor restriction deteriorate the forepaw cutaneous map in the primary somatosensory cortex of adult rats. Exp Brain Res 1999; 129(4):518–531.

[67] Halasi T, Kynsburg A, Tállay A, et al. Changes in joint position sense after surgically treated chronic lateral ankle instability. Br J Sports Med 2005;39(11):818.

[68] Lephart SM, Myers JB, Bradley JP, Fu FH. Shoulder proprioception and function following thermal capsulorrhaphy. Arthroscopy 2002;18 (7):770–778.

[69] Machner A, Wissel H, Heitmann D, Pap G. Changes in proprioceptive capacities of the shoulder joint in ventral shoulder instability. A comparative study before and after arthroscopic labrum refixation. Sportverletz Sportschaden 1998;12(4): 138–141.

[70] Machner A, Merk H, Becker R, Rohkohl K, Wissel H, Pap G. Kinesthetic sense of the shoulder in patients with impingement syndrome. Acta Orthop Scand 2003;74(1):85–88.

[71] Zuckerman JD, Gallagher MA, Cuomo F, Rokito A. The effect of instability and subsequent anterior shoulder repair on proprioceptive ability. J Shoulder Elbow Surg 2003;12(2):105–109.

[72] Xerri C, Merzenich MM, Peterson BE, et al. Plasticity of primary somatosensory cortex paralleling sensorimotor skill recovery from stroke in adult monkeys. J Neurophysiol 1998; 79(4):2119–2148.

[73] Jerosch J, Prymka M. Proprioceptive capacity of the knee joint area in patients after rupture of the anterior cruciate ligament. Unfallchirurg 1996; 99(11):861–868.

[74] Jerosch J, Pfaff G, Thorwesten L, et al. Effects of a proprioceptive training program on sensorimotor capacities of the lower extremity in patients with anterior cruciate ligament instability. Sportverletz Sportschaden 1998;12 (4):121–130.

[75] Jerosch J, Thorwesten L. Proprioceptive abilities of patients with post-traumatic instability of the glenohumeral joint. Z Orthop Ihre Grenzgeb 1998;136(3):230–237.

[76] Roberts D, Friden T, Stomberg A, et al. Bilateral proprioceptive defects in patients with a unilateral anterior cruciate ligament reconstruction: a comparison between patients and healthy individuals. J Orthop Res 2000;18(4):565–571.

[77] Rossi A, Decchi B, Groccia V, et al. Interactions between nociceptive and non-nociceptive afferent projections to cerebral cortex in humans. Neurosci Lett 1998;248(3):155–158.

[78] Weerakkody NS, Blouin JS, Taylor JL, Gandevia SC. Local subcutaneous and muscle pain impairs detection of passive movements at the human thumb. J Physiol 2008;586 (13):3183–3193 Epub 2008 May 8.

[79] Matre D, Arendt-Nielsen L, Knardahl S. Effects of localization and intensity of experimental muscle pain on ankle joint proprioception. Eur J Pain 2002; 6(4):245–260.

[80] Vaillant J, Meunier D, Caillat-Miousse JL. Impact of nociceptive stimuli on cervical kinesthesia. Ann Readapt Med Phys 2008;51(4):257–262 Epub 2008 Apr 29.

[81] Blouin JS, Corbeil P, Teasdale N. Postural stability is altered by the stimulation of pain but not warm receptors in humans.

BMC Musculoskelet Disord 2003;4:23.

[82] Friden T, Roberts D, Ageberg E, et al. Review of knee proprioception and the relation to extremity function after an anterior cruciate ligament rupture. J Orthop Sports Phys Ther 2001;31(10):567–576.

[83] Iguchi Y, Hoshi Y, Hashimoto I. Selective spatial attention induces short-term plasticity in human somatosensory cortex. Neuroreport 2001;12(14): 3133–3136.

[84] Iguchi Y, Hoshi Y, Tanosaki M, et al. Selective attention regulates spatial and intensity information processing in the human primary somatosensory cortex. Neuroreport 2002;13(17): 2335–2339.

[85] Johansen-Berg H, Christensen V, Woolrich M, Matthews PM. Attention to touch modulates activity in both primary and secondary somatosensory areas. Neuroreport 2000;11(6): 1237–1241.

[86] Rushworth MF, Johansen-Berg H, Göbel SM, Devlin JT. The left parietal and premotor cortices: motor attention and selection. Neuroimage 2003;20(Suppl. 1): S89–S100.

[87] Staines WR, Graham SJ, Black SE, McIlroy WE. Task-relevant modulation of contralateral and ipsilateral primary somatosensory cortex and the role of a prefrontal-cortical sensory gating system. Neuroimage 2002;15 (1):190–199.

[88] Flor H, Braun C, Elbert T, Birbaumer N. Extensive reorganization of primary somatosensory cortex in chronic back pain patients. Neurosci Lett 1997;224(1):5–8.

[89] Kempermann G, van Praag H, Gage FH. Activity-dependent regulation of neuronal plasticity and self repair. Prog Brain Res 2000;127:35–48.

[90] Kozorovitskiy Y, Gould E. Adult neurogenesis: a mechanism for brain repair? J Clin Exp Neuropsychol 2003;25(5): 721–732.

[91] Kuhn HG, Palmer TD, Fuchs E. Adult neurogenesis: a compensatory mechanism for neuronal damage. Eur Arch Psych Clin Neurosci 2001;251(4): 152–158.

[92] Peterson DA. Stem cells in brain plasticity and repair. Curr Opin Pharmacol 2002;2(1):34–42.

[93] Pineiro R, Pendlebury S, Johansen-Berg H, Matthews PM. Functional MRI detects posterior shifts in primary sensorimotor cortex activation after stroke: evidence of local adaptive reorganization? Stroke 2001;32:1134–1139.

[94] Barker D, Scott JJ. Regeneration and recovery of cat muscle spindles after devascularization. J Physiol 1990;424:27–39.

[95] Costanzo EM, Barry JA, Ribchester RR. Competition at silent synapses in reinnervated skeletal muscle. Nat Neurosci 2000;3(7):694–700.

[96] Wolf JH, English AW. Muscle spindle reinnervation following phenol block. Cells Tissues Organs 2000;166(4):325–329.

[97] Johnson RD, Munson JB. Regenerating sprouts of axotomized cat muscle afferents express characteristic firing patterns to mechanical stimulation. J Neurophysiol 1991;66(6):2155–2158.

[98] Matsumoto DE, Baker JH. Degeneration and alteration of axons and intrafusal muscle fibres in spindles following tenotomy. Exp Neurol 1987;97:482–498.

[99] Mytskan BM, Mel'man EP. Morphometric characteristics of neuromuscular spindles in hypertrophied skeletal muscle. Biull Eksp Biol Med 1986; 102(11):615–618.

[100] Vrbova MCI, Westbury DR. The sensory reinnervation of hind limb muscles of the cat following denervation and de-efferentation. Neuroscience 1977;2:423–434.

[101] Molteni R, Zheng JQ, Ying Z, et al. Voluntary exercise increases axonal regeneration from sensory neurons. Proc Natl Acad Sci USA 2004;101(22): 8473–8478.

[102] Refshauge KM, Taylor JL, McCloskey DI, et al. Movement detection at the human big toe. J Physiol 1998;513(Part 1): 307–314.

[103] Leinonen V, Kankaanpää M, Luukkonen M, et al. Lumbar paraspinal muscle function, perception of lumbar position, and postural control in disc herniation-related back pain. Spine 2003;28(8):842–848.

[104] Lederman E. The science and practice of manual therapy. London: Elsevier; 2005.

[105] Kennedy JC, Weinberg HW, Wilson AS. The anatomy and function of the anterior cruciate ligament as determined by clinical and morphological studies. J Bone Joint Surg 1974;56:223–235.

[106] Kennedy JC, Alexander IJ, Hayes KC. Nerve supply of the human knee and its functional importance. Am J Sports Med 1982;10:329–335.

[107] Wall JT, Kaas JH, Sur M, et al. Functional reorganization in somatosensory cortical areas 3b and 1 of adult monkeys after median nerve repair: possible relationships to sensory recovery in humans. J Neurosci 1986; 6(1):218–233.

[108] Johansen-Berg H, Dawes H, Guy C, Smith SM, Wade DT, Matthews PM. Correlation between motor improvements and altered fMRI activity after rehabilitative therapy. Brain 2002;125(Part 12):2731–2742.

[109] Zehr PE. Training-induced adaptive plasticity in human somatosensory reflex pathways. J Appl Physiol 2006;101: 1783–1794.

[110] Hurkmans EJ, van der Esch M, Ostelo RW, et al. Reproducibility of the measurement of knee joint proprioception in patients with osteoarthritis of the knee. Arthritis Rheum 2007;57(8): 1398–1403.

[111] Herzog W, Longino D, Clark A. The role of muscles in joint adaptation and degeneration. Langenbecks Arch Surg 2003;388(5):305–315.

[112] Löfvenberg R, Kärrholm J, Lund B. The outcome of nonoperated patients with chronic lateral instability of the ankle: a 20-year follow-up study. Foot Ankle Int 1994; 15(4):165–169.

[113] Chong RK, Ambrose A, Carzoli J, et al. Source of improvement in balance control after a training program for ankle proprioception. Percept Mot Skills 2001;92(1):265–272.

[114] Bernier JN, Perrin DH. Effect of coordination training on proprioception of the functionally unstable ankle. J Orthop Sports Phys Ther 1998;27(4):264–275.

[115] Carter ND, Jenkinson TR, Wilson D, et al. Joint position sense and rehabilitation in the anterior cruciate ligament deficient knee. Br J Sports Med 1997;31(3):209–212.

[116] Holme E, Magnusson SP, Becher K, et al. The effect of supervised rehabilitation on strength, postural sway, position sense and re-injury risk after acute ankle ligament sprain. Scand J Med Sci Sports 1999; 9(2):104–109.

[117] Kynsburg A, Halasi T, Tállay A, et al. Changes in joint position sense after conservatively treated chronic lateral ankle instability. Knee Surg Sports Traumatol Arthrosc 2006; 14(12):1299–1306.

[118] Eils E, Rosenbaum D. A multi-station proprioceptive exercise program in patients with ankle instability. Med Sci Sports Exerc 2001;33(12):1991–1998.

[119] Jan MH, Tang PF, Lin JJ, et al. Efficacy of a target-matching foot-stepping exercise on proprioception and function in patients with knee

osteoarthritis. J Orthop Sports Phys Ther 2008;38(1):19–25.

[120] Rogol IM, Ernst G, Perrin DH. Open and closed kinetic chain exercises improve shoulder joint reposition sense equally in healthy subjects. J Athl Train 1998;33(4):315–318.

[121] Sekir U, Yildiz Y, Hazneci B, et al. Effect of isokinetic training on strength, functionality and proprioception in athletes with functional ankle instability. Knee Surg Sports Traumatol Arthrosc 2007;15(5):654–664.

[122] Thompson KR, Mikesky AE, Bahamonde RE, et al. Effects of physical training on proprioception in older women. J Musculoskelet Neuronal Interact 2003;3(3):223–231.

[123] Swanik KA, Lephart SM, Swanik CB, et al. The effects of shoulder plyometric training on proprioception and selected muscle performance characteristics. J Shoulder Elbow Surg 2002;11 (6):579–586.

[124] Xu D, Hong Y, Li J, et al. Effect of tai chi exercise on proprioception of ankle and knee joints in old people. Br J Sports Med 2004;38(1):50–54.

[125] Li JX, Xu DQ, Hong Y. Tai Chi exercise and proprioception behavior in old people. Med Sport Sci 2008;52:77–86.

[126] Rozzi SL, Lephart SM, Sterner R, et al. Balance training for persons with functionally unstable ankles. J Orthop Sports Phys Ther 1999;29(8):478–486.

[127] Ashton-Miller JA, Wojtys EM, Huston LJ. Can proprioception really be improved by exercises? Knee Surg, Sports Traumatol, Arthrosc 2001;9:128–136.

[128] Handoll HH, Rowe BH, Quinn KM, et al. Interventions

for preventing ankle ligament injuries. Cochrane Database Syst Rev 2001;(3) CD000018.

[129] Paillard J, Brouchon M. Active and passive movements in the calibration of position sense. In: Freedman SJ, editor. The neuropsychology of spatially oriented behavior. Homewood, IL: Dorsey Press; 1968. p. 37–55.

[130] Laufer Y, Hocherman S, Dickstein R. Accuracy of reproducing hand position when using active compared with passive movement. Physiother Res Int 2001;6(2): 65–75.

[131] Lemon RN, Porter R. Short-latency peripheral afferent inputs to pyramidal and other neurons in the precentral cortex of conscious monkeys. In: Gordon G, editor. Active touch. Oxford: Pergamon Press; 1978. p. 91–103.

[132] Gandevia SC, McCloskey DI. Joint sense, muscle sense and their combination as position sense, measured at the distal interphalangeal joint of the middle finger. J Physiol 1976;260:387–407.

[133] Lloyd AJ, Caldwell LS. Accuracy of active and passive positioning of the leg on the basis of kinesthetic cues. J Comp Physiol Psychol 1965; 60(1):102–106.

[134] Friemert B, Bach C, Schwarz W, et al. Benefits of active motion for joint position sense. Knee Surg Sports Traumatol Arthrosc 2006;14(6):564–570.

[135] Silfies SP, Cholewicki J, Reeves NP, Greene HS. Lumbar position sense and the risk of low back injuries in college athletes: a prospective cohort study. BMC Musculoskelet Disord 2007,31;8:129.

Motor adaptation

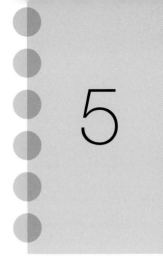

5

Every day we take actions that result in movement and behaviour changes. This can be the consequence of being exposed to new experiences, learning a new task or recovering motor losses after an injury. However, we clearly don't retain all that we have experienced. We seem to remember or learn only certain events. Some physical actions become our movement repertoire, while others seem to disappear in time. Similarly, how can we be certain that rehabilitation will result in effective and lasting motor changes?

To answer this question we need to examine how we naturally attain lifelong motor changes. It seems that there are certain factors within our behaviour that are important for facilitating adaptation in the neuromuscular system. These factors can be viewed as a form of code for neuromuscular adaptation. Rehabilitation programmes that contain these code elements are more likely to be effective in recovering motor losses and promoting long-term motor and behavioural changes.

The code for neuromuscular adaptation

The neuromuscular adaptation code elements can be identified by observing a person's behaviour during a motor learning situation. For example, in order to learn to play the piano the individual has to be aware of the score, the relationship of the keys to the scales, placement of the hand on the keys and so on. It involves physical, active practice at the keyboard. The person will continuously monitor their

mistakes and correct them; often playing the same scales in numerous repetitions. Furthermore, we are intuitively aware that lifting weights at the gym will not improve playing the piano. In order to play the piano one has to practise playing the piano. From this example five basic adaptation code elements can be identified (Fig. 5.1):

1. Cognition
2. Being active
3. Feedback
4. Repetition
5. Similarity principle.

It should be noted that motor learning and adaptation share the same neurophysiological mechanisms.[1] However, rehabilitation following musculoskeletal injuries or pain conditions is not about learning a novel motor pattern. Most patients are fully aware of what movement they have to perform but are unable to physically carry it out. Their inability is often due to a mix of physical losses and an underlying motor reorganization or dysfunction (Chs 9–12).

Adaptive code 1: cognition

In the context of neuromuscular rehabilitation cognition is the mental process in which the patient is aware of and attentive to the movement experience, understands its aims and goals, and is able to make decisions and organize a response. It is also the process of thinking, rationalizing and memorizing.

The role of cognition in neuromuscular rehabilitation can be demonstrated by an example. A fell

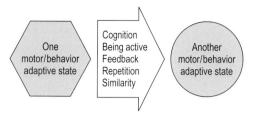

Fig. 5.1 • Experiences that contain the five code elements are more like to promote adaptive changes within the neuromuscular system resulting in movement and behavioural changes.

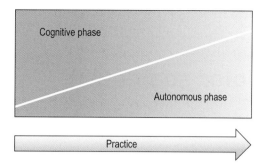

Fig. 5.2 • The transition from cognitive to autonomous phase during motor learning. Throughout the transition some elements will remain cognitive and autonomous.

runner who trained on rough terrain found that she was tripping with increasing regularity. Consequently she began to train on flat paved surfaces. She was aware that something had changed in her control, but could not understand her progressive inability. During challenged balance she demonstrated gross postural control losses that were later linked to recurrent severe bilateral ankle sprains. Patients often experience such progressive deterioration of performance without being able to understand their underlying causes and, consequently, how to rectify them. The role of cognition in this case was to inform the patient about her condition, bring attention to the specific losses and work out, with the patient, a management that would challenge these losses.

Neuromuscular rehabilitation is about changes in motor patterns or movement behaviour. Cognition is a potent modifier of behaviour and, therefore, of motor control. A change in movement behaviour can be as simple as bringing attention to the way a person performs a movement and correcting it verbally or by demonstration. For example, a teenage tennis player developed medial knee pain over a period of several weeks. It was brought to his attention that this injury could be related to a movement pattern which exerted a medial stress on the knee. He immediately recognized a newly acquired side-stepping pattern in which he would adduct and drag the non-weight-bearing leg on the ground. He also knew the solution (not to do it) and was aware how to implement the change. He required no further treatment and rapidly recovered from the injury (see Task-behaviour sphere, Ch. 8). The whole management took place within the cognitive dimension.

Cognition and phases of learning

We all have the experience that when we practise a new movement after a while we don't have to think how to carry it out: it seems to occur just by "wanting" to do it. This phenomenon represents a phase in motor learning where there is a transition from a *cognitive phase* to a subconscious *autonomous phase* (Fig. 5.2).[2]

The early, cognitive stages of learning are characterized by the high levels of intellectual activity needed to understand the meaning of the information, the nature of the task and how to refine it. The individual may be aware of doing something wrong, but they are incapable of fully understanding and improving it.[2]

As the individual becomes more proficient in performing a skill, it becomes more "automatic" and less under conscious control. In this phase, the skill is stored as a motor programme and becomes more robust to interference from other ongoing activities and environmental disturbances. Hence, in the cognitive phase it may be more difficult to multitask, whereas this becomes easier in the autonomous phase.[2] Autonomous activity is not totally subconscious and some elements of the movement will remain in the individual's awareness (Fig. 5.3).[2]

The transition between the two learning phases can often be observed in rehabilitation. Initially, the patient will perform a movement that is inaccurate and requires intense concentration. After several sessions the movement patterns become more skilled and subconscious. The hallmark of the transition into the autonomous phase is when the patient is no longer attentive to the movement and is able to multitask, e.g. simultaneously conversing with the therapist. This should be encouraged as it may help to facilitate the transition into the autonomous state.[3]

Often a dysfunctional movement may become the habitual autonomous pattern. For example, some patients may be unaware of the compensatory/coping

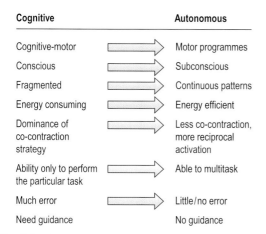

Cognitive		Autonomous
Cognitive-motor	⟹	Motor programmes
Conscious	⟹	Subconscious
Fragmented	⟹	Continuous patterns
Energy consuming	⟹	Energy efficient
Dominance of co-contraction strategy	⟹	Less co-contraction, more reciprocal activation
Ability only to perform the particular task	⟹	Able to multitask
Much error	⟹	Little/no error
Need guidance		No guidance

Fig. 5.3 • Some features of the cognitive and autonomous phases.

strategies they use to compensate for control losses.[4] In these situations the motor dysfunction is transferred into the autonomous phase and becomes resistant to change. To reverse this, the patient needs to be brought back to the cognitive phase and retrained in the correct movement pattern (see Task behaviour sphere, Ch. 8). Once they are able to execute the movement correctly, the rehabilitation would aim to assist its transition back to the autonomous state.

> ### Clinical note
>
> Generally, the aim of neuromuscular rehabilitation is to bring motor control to an autonomous state where it becomes part of the habitual movement repertoire.

"Active cognition" and "passive cognition"

There is a common experience that when we are driven as a passenger to a new address we may find it difficult to remember the route. However, having to actively learn the route tends to improve the memory of it.

There seems to be a difference in learning between being "actively" or "passively" aware. Subjects tend to learn a motor task more effectively when they are given more choice over how to practise and how much feedback to receive ("active cognition").[5] If they are given a pre-organized blocked training programme and predetermined feedback

they tend not to learn the movement as well ("passive-cognitive"). This phenomenon has been demonstrated in maze training. One group received training that restricted their movements to the correct path, so that no choice was made (passively-cognitive). Another group was given choices while moving through the maze (actively-cognitive).[6] The maze learning of the "choice" group was greatly superior to that of the "no-choice" group, although both forms of guidance were cognitive.

> ### Clinical note
>
> Motor learning could be optimized by enabling the patients to make decisions and enabling them to have control over the scheduling and sequencing during rehabilitation.[7]

Selective attention and memories of doing

During rehabilitation patients are often guided to focus on the particulars of their movement or goals of their actions. This focus (*selective attention*) helps the sensory-motor system to adapt and modify our behaviour.[8] Events which are out of attention will often be forgotten over time. In some remarkable way attention drives sensory-motor adaptation. The analogy is in listening to music and remembering only the melody line played by the lead instrument. Although we can hear all the other instruments, only the ones we focus on can be remembered. This phenomenon can be observed in (blind) Braille readers. The selective focus on their reading index finger results in specific enlargement of the finger's cortical representation.[9]

Generally, there is a limited ability to focus on more than one stream of information or actions at a time (try reading the next paragraph and count backwards from ten to zero).[10-12] In musculoskeletal conditions pain itself may become the focus of attention and, therefore, competes with other attention demands.[10]

Internal and external focus and learning

When walking across a room full of strangers most individuals have had the experience of becoming very aware of their own body and movement. As this happens, momentarily, we don't know what to do with our arms and the whole process of walking seems to become more awkward and less skilled. This experience may be due to a phenomenon that occurs when there is a shift of attention from the goal of movement to the details of how to do it.

When the focus of attention is directed to the goals of the movement it is termed *external focus*. When the focus is on the internal workings of the body or the details of the action it is often referred to as *internal focus*.[5] During the early phase of learning attention is drawn internally to the particulars of the action – the technique, the position of the hand; the pressure used, etc.[13] This focus shifts externally as the individual becomes more skilled in performing the movement.

For a skilled person, learning improves if training uses external focus directed to the goals of the movements rather than to the details of the actions. For example, there is greater accuracy in tennis serves and football shots when the subjects use external-focus rather than internal-focus strategies.[14,15] Conversely, skilled performance can degrade if an internal focus is used, such as focusing on the hand during tennis serves.[5,16] Even conscious tensing of the trunk muscle (internal focus) has been shown to degrade postural control.[17]

The use of internal and external focus during rehabilitation may depend on whether the patient is an "unskilled injured" or "skilled injured". The unskilled injured is a novice who in the process of acquiring/learning their skills has been injured. In this scenario, rehabilitation should comprise internal- and external-focus principles, since the patient still has to learn the novel movement, which requires some internal focus. In contrast, the "skilled injured" are experienced in the task, but are physically unable to perform it. An external-focus approach may be more beneficial for this group since they don't have to learn the movement from scratch.

This does not exclude the use of both focusing approaches for the "injured skilled". Skilled movements degrade over time, especially if the individual has been unable to perform normal movements due to a long-term injury – a sort of "motor forgetting".[18] This can be seen in patients who walk with a limp long after they have recovered from their injury. In this condition, it may be helpful to revert temporarily to an internal-focus approach, drawing attention to the particulars of the walking cycle, such as the heel strike. Internal focus strategies may be also be beneficial for patients with central

nervous system (CNS) damage.[19] (Although in my clinic I found that I tend to gravitate away from using internal focus with CNS-damaged patients).[19,20]

It has been shown that the focus of attention during learning is different in children and adults.[21] Children tend to favour internal focus whereas adults tend to focus more externally on the task. The difference could be due to the fact that children are less motorically experienced, whereas adults are able to draw on their previous motor experiences.

Extreme internal and external focus

How far internally can a person afford to focus before it becomes detrimental to learning? Some movement rehabilitation approaches promote internal focusing on particular muscles or muscle chains: a form of "extreme internal focusing". In these approaches the muscle itself becomes the focus or movement goal. For example, in core-stability training transversus abdominis is often the focus of rehabilitation.[22] Also currently in fashion is a focus on the improvement in the efficiency of the scapular stabilizers for shoulder conditions and the enhancement in the control of the deep anterior cervical muscles for patients suffering from chronic neck pain.

In the last decade several studies have examined this issue. In one such study participants performed basketball shots using either internal focus (focus on wrist motion) or external focus (basket).[23] Compared to internal focus, the external group had better accuracy and lower EMG activity of the biceps and triceps muscles. This suggests that an external focus of attention optimizes movement economy.[23]

Even focusing on the effort of the movement (internal) will result in inferior learning when compared to focusing on the goal of the movement (external).[24]

In a study using balance as an outcome measure, participants were instructed to focus their attention on markers which were placed at different distances from their body. It was found that the postural control improved the further away the focus from the body was.[16] In another study, participants balanced on a stabilometer while holding a tube horizontally.[15] In one group the tube was empty while in the other the tube contained a ball that had to be kept central. Participants were instructed to either focus on their hands (internal focus), or on the empty tube (external focus) or on a sort of "super-external" focus on the ball in the tube. In both experiments, the external focus groups demonstrated more effective learning and transfer than the internal focus groups, both in learning the tube-ball skill and the balancing task itself. However, the super-external had the best learning outcomes both in the tube and the balancing tasks. This phenomenon of super-external focus was demonstrated in stroke patients.[25] Two groups of patients trained in walking, but one group had to play with a ball while walking. The group with the extra-external task had greater improvement in walking than the group practising the single task of walking.

More recently this phenomenon was demonstrated in re-training postural stability after lateral ankle sprain. The external focus ("keep your balance by stabilising the platform") was found to be more effective than the internal focus ("keep your balance by stabilising your body").[26] Furthermore, the internal focus group did not improve their balance at all.[27]

Interestingly, Eastern movement traditions, such as tai chi and yoga, often use internal focus strategies for learning and performance of movement. Yet, it was demonstrated that tai chi training improves balance,[28] as well as coordination during gait initiation.[29] It was as effective as functional balance and leg strength exercise (mostly external focus) in reducing the incidents of falling in pre-frail individuals.[30]

Clinical note

Neuromuscular rehabilitation should move away from training approaches that focus attention on specific muscles, muscle chains or joints. Movement should be practised as a whole with an emphasis on external focus and movement goals. This approach is applicable to the majority of patients who receive rehabilitation: they know what to do but can't do it ("skilled injured"). Patients with central motor losses may benefit from a mix of internal- and external-focus strategies.[19,20] Probably, a pragmatic approach is best – see what the patient can cope with or what seems to be more beneficial (constructive tinkering in the face of uncertainty).

Adaptive code 2: being active

Being active and physically practising the movement is essential for neuromuscular adaptation. During active movement, the whole of the motor system is engaged. In contrast, during passive movement, there is no efferent activity or muscle recruitment (see The comparator system, Ch. 2).[31] In order to

learn we need to make mistakes and correct them. Without the efferent/motor component there are no errors to correct and hence little, if any, learning. This has been demonstrated in studies where vision was distorted by special lenses. The ability of the subject to learn to correct arm movement was greatly enhanced by active rather than passive arm movement.[32] Interestingly, passive movement rarely occurs during normal daily activities.[33] It can be inferred from this observation that the motor system is well accustomed to adapt to active rather than passive movement.

These issues of passive versus active approach are important in the context of neuromuscular rehabilitation and manual therapy. There are several disciplines that promote the belief that motor control can be somehow manipulated by passive approaches, for example spinal manipulation to normalize segmental muscle tone.[34–39] Such approaches are likely to produce only brief, reflexive responses.

Facilitating motor learning with mental practice

Despite the apparent need for physical practice, motor learning can be enhanced by mental rehearsal or by a demonstration of a movement (Fig. 5.4).[40,41]

Mental practice has been shown to improve activities such as bowling, piano-playing and ball-throwing (can air-guitarists play real guitars?). Even movement variables such as force, endurance and movement-time have been shown to improve with mental practice.[42–46] It was shown that in weight training the physical practice group improved their

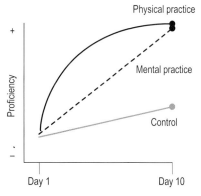

Fig. 5.4 • Mental practice can enhance motor learning. Mental rehearsal of some tasks can be almost as effective as physically practising it. (From: Rawlings EI, Rawlings IL, Chen CS et al 1972 The facilitating effects of mental rehearsal in the acquisition of rotary pursuit tracking. Psychonomic Science 26:71–73.)

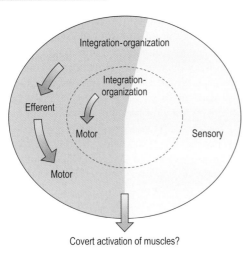

Covert activation of muscles?

Fig. 5.5 • Mental practice activates the efferent/motor component of the motor process. It may involve low-level activation in the muscles associated with the particular task being rehearsed.

strength by 30% while the mental practice group increased it by 20%. This force increase by mental practice is probably due to central motor reorganization of force control rather than muscle hypertrophy.

Mental practice facilitates motor adaptation by activating the motor system in much the same way as physical practice.[12] Imagining a movement activates cortical motor areas in similar patterns to those activated during actual physical practice.[47] It may also engage minimally the muscles that are involved in the imagined task but without producing observable movement. When subjects are asked to visualize hitting a nail with a hammer twice, the electromyograph (EMG) trace demonstrates two separate bursts of activity that are correlated with the imagined movement.[43] A similar process takes place when we mentally recite words. The vocal muscles are minutely activated, although no sound is produced (Fig. 5.5).[43]

In the last few years mental practice has moved from the motor learning to the rehabilitation sphere and was shown to improve motor control in stroke patients.[48,49] This learning strategy may also be useful for patients who have been immobilized or unable to move due to musculoskeletal injuries.[44]

Adaptive code 3: feedback

Since we learn by making mistakes we need feedback to inform us how well we are achieving our movement goals. Feedback can be *intrinsic* from proprioception or *extrinsic* in the form of verbal instructions, visual demonstration or even physical, tactile correction of movement by a therapist/trainer.[12,40,41]

Intrinsic, proprioceptive losses will impair the ability to correct, improve or learn new movement (Ch. 2 & 4).[32,50–54] Under such circumstances the individual will often compensate for this loss by shifting their attention to another sensory source, e.g. to vision if proprioception is lost.

Extrinsic feedback plays an important role in rehabilitation and is often referred to as guidance or *kinaesthetic feedback*.[55] It is often used to provide information about the details and "correctness" of the movement ("hold the racket this way"), the movement sequences ("swing it like this") or the quality in performance ("good shot").

Generally, guidance is more effective if it promotes an active gathering of information and problem-solving by the patient. The outcome is improved motor learning and a wider repertoire of movement responses and learning that transfers readily to other situations.[56] For optimum learning, guidance should be kept to the minimum and should be rapidly reduced or fully withdrawn at the earliest opportunity.[5,11,57,58,59,60]

Young children seem to depend on longer periods of feedback during motor learning.[61] This may be due to their having a limited range of motor experiences on which they can draw when learning.

Adaptive code 4: repetition

We all have had the experience that to master a certain skill we need to put in the practice (Table 5.1).[41] The frequency and the number of repetitions in practising specific tasks will have important implications for the recovery of motor losses. Like a well-trodden path on a grass lawn, actions that are repeated will pave stable and enduring neuronal paths within the CNS.

Repetition together with selective attention plays a crucial role in the transformation of motor experiences from short- to long-term memory. This transformation is a sequential process often described as occurring in three stages; from short-term sensory store to short-term memory and, finally, long-term memory.[2,12,62,63] Once a pattern has been stored in the long-term memory it will not be lost in the absence of rehearsal. Indeed, this can be observed in activities such as swimming, cycling or playing a

Table 5.1 Estimated numbers of repetitions required to achieve skilled performance

Activity	Repetition for skilled performance
Cigar-making	3 million cigars
Hand knitting	1.5 million stitches
Rug-making	1.4 million knots
Violin playing	2.5 million notes
Walking, up to 6 years	3 million steps
Marching	0.8 million steps
Pearl-handling	1.5–3 million
Football passing	1.4 million passes
Basketball playing	1 million baskets
Gymnastics performing	8 years' daily practice

musical instrument, activities that can be recalled after many years without practice.[12]

The meaning and relevance to the individual, motivational factors and the emotional value in the experience also play a part in long-term memory. Generally, experiences with strong personal or emotional significance are more likely to transfer rapidly to long-term memory.[12] The extreme example of this is often seen in individuals who have been in a single traumatic experience, such as a road traffic accident. They may develop long-term sensitization and motor/behavioural changes in the absence of any serious tissue damage.[64]

Repetition and practice of tasks is important throughout the spectrum of neuromuscular conditions seen in clinic.[65] In stroke patients it was demonstrated that repetition can result in positive gains in performance even after one day of training.[66]

Adaptive code 5: similarity principle and transfer

Following injury most individuals will take actions to overcome their losses without any medical intervention. These actions often resemble the movement patterns which they have lost. A person with a sprained ankle, who could not walk, will attempt to walk and, likewise, an injured tennis player will attempt to gradually return to playing tennis. This is nature's "gold standard" for recovery of movement control – practise what you have lost (or what you would like to gain). This natural phenomenon is the basis of the *similarity principle*. It proposes that learning is more effective when the training resembles the task which is being recovered.[40,67] The similarity principle is one of the most important issues in neuromuscular rehabilitation. *It determines which activities or movement patterns will be the focus of treatment.*

It seems that for learning or recovering particular movement patterns the practice should be both **similar and within the context** of the task. This suggests that if a patient cannot balance during walking, rehabilitation should focus on balance during walking.[30,68,69] Equally, if force losses impede stair-climbing, than leg strength should be challenged during that or a very similar activity.[70] If the patient, due to lack of coordination, cannot raise their arm to eat then rehabilitation should focus on coordination within similar movement patterns. Under these circumstances the individual parts of the whole movement are being practised simultaneously, i.e. the *relationships between them* are being rehearsed.[12] Practising movement which is similar and within context is more likely to *transfer* to related daily activities. Transfer is the ability to take a motor experience from one situation and apply it to another.[67,71–73]

Practising a dissimilar movement pattern or movement that is out of context may reduce the likelihood of transfer (Fig. 5.6). Imagine a patient who has standing difficulties due to a balance problem. The treatment will be *dissimilar* if strength exercises, such as standing knee squats, are used to challenge standing balance.[74] The strength challenge is the dissimilar element as it fails to challenge balance. However, it is still performed within the context of standing. The rehabilitation will be out of *context* if the training for balance is practised sitting on a Swiss ball. In this situation the balance is similar but movement is performed whilst sitting and is, therefore, out of the context of standing. The rehabilitation can be both dissimilar and out of context, for example straight leg rising (dissimilar) practised on the floor (out of context).

The importance of similarity and context has been highlighted by several studies. Resistance

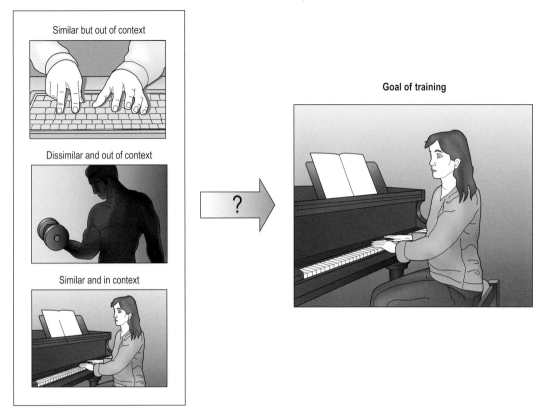

Fig. 5.6 • Similarity and context in rehabilitation.

cycling or seated strength exercise will improve strength in these activities, but have little or no effect on walking for a stroke patient, because strength may not be the control issue here.[75,76] Strength training in sitting may help the patient in getting up;[76] a situation where force may be necessary. However, would not practising getting up be equally, or even more, effective? For stroke patients sitting and reaching training improves sitting and reaching, and the production of vertical force through the leg as they lean forward.[77] The vertical force improvement in the leg seems to transfer to improvement in getting up from the sitting position, but no aspect of that training transfers to walking. However, training of stroke patients in walking improves walking speed and distance, but not balance.[78,79] Balance seems to be improved by challenging balance.[80] But challenging static balance in standing might not transfer well to dynamic balance during walking.[81] Yes, the similarity principle can be that finicky.

How similar should training be?

Current research cannot provide the answer as to how far a treatment can stray from 100% similarity (Fig. 5.7). The studies in motor control and learning are very adamant that it should be very close.[12] However, most of these studies have been carried out on healthy individuals who are learning new and unfamiliar tasks. As discussed previously, neuromuscular rehabilitation involves individuals who are not true learners; they are being retrained in activities that they have experienced in the past. They are "readjusting" rather than learning something new.

We can imagine 100% should give the best result. If walking is affected then just practise walking. However, in the case of a patient who is unable to execute 100% similarity, how far can they afford to stray from that ideal and still improve? For example, I have been working with a stroke patient who was unable to walk, partly due to inability to flex

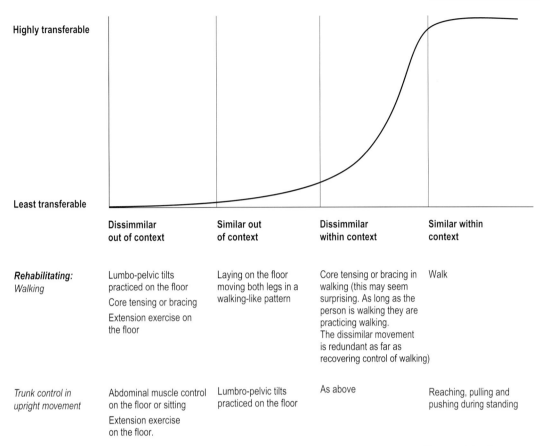

	Dissimmilar out of context	Similar out of context	Dissimmilar within context	Similar within context
Rehabilitating: *Walking*	Lumbo-pelvic tilts practiced on the floor Core tensing or bracing Extension exercise on the floor	Laying on the floor moving both legs in a walking-like pattern	Core tensing or bracing in walking (this may seem surprising. As long as the person is walking they are practicing walking. The dissimilar movement is redundant as far as recovering control of walking)	Walk
Trunk control in upright movement	Abdominal muscle control on the floor or sitting Extension exercise on the floor.	Lumbro-pelvic tilts practiced on the floor	As above	Reaching, pulling and pushing during standing

Fig. 5.7 • How similar is your rehabilitation? The effectiveness of practice can be assessed by examining how similar it is and whether it is in the context of the goals of training. Rehabilitation is likely to be more effective if it is similar and within the context of the movement goals of the treatment.

the hypertonic extended knee. We proceeded to improve this movement in sitting. After a long and intense focusing on this particular movement the patient regained the ability to flex and extend the knee, as well as execute rhythmic pendular movements (similar but out of context to walking). It would be logical to assume that once it has been mastered, the patient should be able to transfer the control of knee bending to walking. This was a humiliating lesson in similarity and transfer. It had absolutely no effect on bending the knee during standing. It was as if he had never practised that movement at all.

It is difficult to identify how close the training should be to the goal of rehabilitation. The simple solution is to endeavour to keep the training close to the 100% similarity and in context; unless the patient is unable to perform similar movement patterns or execute them within context.

Is recovery transferrable?

Imagine a patient who has a balance/postural stability problem. We would expect that all upright, weight-bearing activities that depend on balance will be affected. Is the reverse also true? Would balance training during standing or walking transfer to running, skipping climbing stairs or playing basketball?

We can only *assume* that recovery in balance/ postural stability in one or two weight-bearing activities (walking, stairs) will also improve all other related upright activities (running, hopping on a tennis court). If this assumption is correct it provides an interesting therapeutic shortcut. There is no need to rehabilitate every physical action in a person's movement repertoire. All that may be needed is to "re-abilitate" the specific abilities which are shared by several skills. This assumption

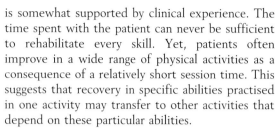

is somewhat supported by clinical experience. The time spent with the patient can never be sufficient to rehabilitate every skill. Yet, patients often improve in a wide range of physical activities as a consequence of a relatively short session time. This suggests that recovery in specific abilities practised in one activity may transfer to other activities that depend on these particular abilities.

The transfer of training can be in two directions: a "lateral" and a "vertical" transfer. A lateral transfer would be to similar tasks, such as from walking to stair-climbing. A vertical transfer is the same task but at increased difficulty (greater force, amplitude, speed, range, etc.).[82–85] Walking with a rucksack which increases the load is a vertical transfer. It requires complex neuromuscular reorganization compared to free walking, but does not require any extra learning.[86]

Lateral and vertical transfer was demonstrated in a study examining the effects of exercise on neuromuscular control after knee menisscectomy. The patients presented with neuromuscular deficits and functional limitations, which were evident several years after their operation. The exercise programme comprised postural stability training and functional strength and endurance exercises for leg and trunk muscles. The exercise group showed significant improvement in hamstrings strength and quadriceps endurance (vertical transfer), but, importantly, they also improved in one-leg hop, something they did not train for (lateral transfer). There is also evidence that training in tai chi transfers laterally to postural stability and coordination.[87] Another example of vertical transfer was shown in subjects with lateral ankle sprain. It was demonstrated that training under moderately unstable conditions can transfer to improvements in postural control under more challenging stability conditions.[27]

Inter-limb transfer: the left hand does know what the right hand is doing!

Learning a task on one side of the body can sometimes transfer to the other side.[88,89] For example, strength training on one side was shown to transfer to the opposite side (about a 10% increase).[90] This could be due to the motor programmes being a generalized scheme of movement rather than being limb-specific (Ch. 2). Interestingly, brain scans demonstrate that motor learning on one side of the body tends to bring about similar cortical changes in both hemispheres.[91]

Movement strategies in painful conditions may also transfer to the opposite limb; probably through the same central mechanisms. In patients with chronic wrist pain, coordination losses were evident in the affected and, to a lesser extent, in the non-affected hand.[92]

There may also be a sensory transfer between the two limbs. In individuals who had cruciate ligament reconstruction or shoulder injury, decreased proprioceptive ability was present in some measurements in the injured as well as the uninjured side.[93,94]

The clinical implication of this inter-limb transfer is not clear. It is yet to be established whether treating the non-injured limb will result in significant clinical improvement of the injured limb (I am placing my bets on treating the injured limb).

Variability in training

The similarity principle suggests that training should be as close as possible to the goal movement. However, most movement patterns are highly variable. In the clinic often the variability is reflected in changing the movement parameters or varying the task itself. During the rehabilitation of walking, variability would reflect in practising different walking speeds or stride lengths. Furthermore, walking itself can be practised in different tasks: walk sideways, walk over an obstacle, stairs, heel-toe, walk and turn, and any other variation. From studies of healthy subjects and individuals suffering from central damage, such variability during training helps to improve retention and transfer and increases the movement repertoire.[12,30,40,95,96,97]

Different tasks can be introduced in various sequences. *Blocked practice* is when each task is practised individually, for example walking only. Another possibility is to mix several related tasks in random practice,[12,95] for example walking, stairs, running, skipping, etc. Generally, a more random sequence seems to be beneficial for individuals with an intact CNS.[95,96,98] This form of practice introduces greater cognitive/motor processing demands on the individual. It tends to reduce performance during the training/treatment sessions but seems to benefit retention and transfer (which is the important bit).

Patients suffering from CNS conditions, such as Alzheimer's and Parkinson's disease, where cognitive demands can be an issue, seem to do better in retention and transfer when the tasks are practised individually and repetitively.[99,100,101] Clinically, a pragmatic approach is probably useful for scheduling of tasks. Use the patterns that the patient can cope with, rather than using a strict protocol.

Neuromuscular exercises – do they exist?

There is a trend to label some forms of training as neuromuscular exercise.[102,103] Is there such a distinct training entity? All exercises performed actively by the patient are neuromuscular. Whether they are performed lying down, sitting or with the aid of machines; they are all challenging the neuromuscular system. Presumably, what is meant is that some exercises are more within the context of certain sports or related tasks. Hence, they are more functional to that particular athlete and their sports. This is in contrast to exercises such as the traditional force training in the gym, which are dissimilar, out of context and may even be extra-functional.

Is one approach better in some way? The very few studies that do exist generally demonstrate better outcome in various measures for the functional exercise (neuromuscular exercise) compared with more traditional strength training.[68,104] However, it seems that functional training may bring about additional motor control benefits. For example, standing balance training can give the same strength gain in the leg as using specific machines for leg curls and leg presses.[68] The balance training had the further advantage of improving balance and equalising the muscle forces between the dominant and non-dominant leg.[68] Hence, exercises that are similar and within context are more likely to challenge a greater range of underlying abilities, including the composite abilities, such as balance/postural stability, single, multi-limb and whole body coordination.

Summary points

- For effective motor adaptation/learning, the practice needs to employ five principal elements: cognition, being active, feedback, repetition and similarity.
- Cognitive: the patient should be attentive to their movement and encouraged to process and make decisions about their actions.
- Active: being physically active is important for motor learning. Passive approaches are unlikely to be effective in promoting lasting and functional motor control changes. Mental practice, an active cognitive process, activates the whole motor system and, therefore, may be a valuable clinical tool.
- Feedback can be intrinsic from proprioception or extrinsic, such as guidance by the therapist.
- Repetition, repetition, repetition – very important for long-term memory.
- Similarity: rehabilitation should use movement patterns that are similar to and within the context of the movement being recovered.
- Rehabilitation which is dissimilar or out of context is unlikely to transfer from the session to daily activities.

Table 5.2 Differences in motor learning strategies between young children and adults

Young	Adults
Observing, mimicking, some cognition?	Use cognition
Favour internal focus	Favour external focus
Cope better with less variability in practice	Favour variability
Need more feedback	Minimal feedback
Greater need for repetition	Need repetition but not as much
May require longer rehabilitation due to lack of motor experience ("unskilled injured")	Know the movement but can't perform it ("skilled injured") Motor re-adaptation and reorganization rather than true learning

- Experiences that possess a higher content of adaptive code elements have a greater potential for promoting long-term changes.
- Experiences with low code content will fail to promote any significant adaptation and will result in an ineffective, short-lived response to treatment.
- External focus is more effective for motor learning. Internal focus should be used only in learning novel movements or if the

patient has "forgotten" how to move correctly. Internal focus should be withdrawn as soon as the patient is able to perform the movement.

- Internal focus approach may be more beneficial for patients with CNS conditions.
- Children and adults may use different motor learning strategies which may influence the treatment approach (Table 5.2).
- Air guitarists can't play real guitars.

References

[1] Winstein C, Wing AM, Whitall. Motor control and learning principles for rehabilitation of upper limb movement after brain injury. In: Grafman J, Robertson IH, editors. Handbook of neuropsychology, vol. 9. 2nd ed. London: Elsevier; 2003.

[2] Magill RA. Motor learning concepts and applications. Iowa: William C Brown; 1985.

[3] Karni A, Meyer G, Rey-Hipolito C, et al. The acquisition of skilled motor performance: fast and slow experience-driven changes in primary motor cortex. Proc Natl Acad Sci USA 1998;95(3):861–868.

[4] Cameron M, Adams R, Maher C. Motor control and strength as predictors of hamstring injury in elite players of Australian football. Phys Ther Sport 2004;4(4):159–166.

[5] McNevin NH, Wulf G, Carlson C. Effects of attentional focus, self-control, and dyad training on motor learning: implications for physical rehabilitation. Phys Ther 2000;80(4):373–385.

[6] Von-Wright JM. A note on the role of guidance in learning. Br J Psychol 1957;48:133–137.

[7] Seidler RD. Multiple motor learning experiences enhance motor adaptability. J Cogn Neurosci 2004;16(1):65–73.

[8] Kahneman D. Attention and effort. Englewood Cliffs: Prentice Hall; 1973.

[9] Pascual-Leone A, Cohen LG, Hallet M. Cortical map plasticity in humans. Trends Neurosci 1992;15(1):13–14.

[10] Lamoth CJ, Stins JF, Pont M, et al. Effects of attention on the control of locomotion in individuals with chronic low back pain. J Neuroeng Rehabil 2008;5:13.

[11] Schmidt RA, Wulf G. Continuous concurrent feedback degrades skill learning: implications for training and simulation. Hum Factors 1997;39(4):509–525.

[12] Schmidt RA, Lee TD. Motor control and learning. 4th ed. UK: Human Kinetics; 2005.

[13] Beilock SL, Carr TH, MacMahon C, Starkes JL. When paying attention becomes counterproductive: impact of divided versus skill-focused attention on novice and experienced performance of sensorimotor skills. J Exp Psychol Appl 2002;8(1):6–16.

[14] Wulf G, McConnel N, Gärtner M, Schwarz A. Enhancing the learning of sport skills through external-focus feedback. J Mot Behav 2002;34(2):171–182.

[15] Wulf G, Weigelt M, Poulter D, McNevin N. Attentional focus on suprapostural tasks affects balance learning. Q J Exp Psychol A. 2003;56(7):1191–1211.

[16] McNevin NH, Shea CH, Wulf G. Increasing the distance of an external focus of attention enhances learning. Psychol Res 2003;67(1):22–29.

[17] Reeves NP, Everding VQ, Cholewicki J, Morrisette DC. The effects of trunk stiffness on postural control during unstable

seated balance. Exp Brain Res 2006;174(4):694–700.

[18] Punt TD, Riddoch MJ. Motor neglect: implications for movement and rehabilitation following stroke. Disabil Rehabil 2006;28(13–14):857–864.

[19] Cirstea MC, Levin MF. Improvement of arm movement patterns and endpoint control depends on type of feedback during practice in stroke survivors. Neurorehabil Neural Repair 2007;21(5):398–411.

[20] van Vliet PM, Wulf G. Extrinsic feedback for motor learning after stroke: what is the evidence? Disabil Rehabil 2006;28 (13–14):831–840.

[21] Emanuel M, Jarus T, Bart O. Effect of focus of attention and age on motor acquisition, retention, and transfer: a randomized trial. Phys Ther 2008;88(2):251–260 . Epub 2007 Nov 27.

[22] O'Sullivan PB. Lumbar segmental 'instability': clinical presentation and specific stabilizing exercise management. Man Ther 2000;5(1):2–12.

[23] Zachry T, Wulf G, Mercer J, et al. Increased movement accuracy and reduced EMG activity as the result of adopting an external focus of attention. Brain Res Bull 2005;67(4): 304–309.

[24] Kurtzer I, DiZio P, Lackner J. Task-dependent motor learning. Exp Brain Res 2003;153(1):128–132.

[25] Yang YR, Wang RY, Chen YC, et al. Dual-task exercise improves walking ability in chronic stroke: a

randomized controlled trial. Arch Phys Med Rehabil 2007;88(10):1236–1240.

[26] Laufer Y, Rotem-Lehrer N, Ronen Z, et al. Effect of attention focus on acquisition and retention of postural control following ankle sprain. Arch Phys Med Rehabil 2007;88(1):105–108.

[27] Rotem-Lehrer N, Laufer Y. Effect of focus of attention on transfer of a postural control task following an ankle sprain. J Orthop Sports Phys Ther 2007;37(9):564–569.

[28] Taylor-Piliae RE, Haskell WL, Stotts NA, et al. Improvement in balance, strength, and flexibility after 12 weeks of Tai chi exercise in ethnic Chinese adults with cardiovascular disease risk factors. Altern Ther Health Med 2006;12(2):50–58.

[29] Hass CJ, Gregor RJ, Waddell DE, et al. The influence of Tai Chi training on the center of pressure trajectory during gait initiation in older adults. Arch Phys Med Rehabil 2004; 85(10):1593–1598.

[30] Faber MJ, Bosscher RJ, Chin A, Paw MJ, et al. Effects of exercise programs on falls and mobility in frail and pre-frail older adults: A multicenter randomized controlled trial. Arch Phys Med Rehabil 2006;87(7):885–896.

[31] Ralston HJ, Libet B. The question of tonus in skeletal muscles. Am J Phys Med 1953;32:85–92.

[32] Held R. Plasticity in sensorimotor coordination. In: Freedman SJ, editor. The neuropsychology of spatially oriented behavior. Homewood, IL: Dorsey Press; 1968.

[33] Matthews PBC. Proprioceptors and their contribution to somatosensory mapping: complex messages require complex processing. Can J Physiol Pharmacol 1988;66:430–438.

[34] Herzog W, Scheele D, Conway PJ. Electromyographic responses of back and limb muscles associated with spinal manipulative therapy. Spine 1999;24(2):146–152.

[35] Pickar JG, Wheeler JD. Response of muscle proprioceptors to spinal manipulative-like loads in the anesthetized cat. J Manipulative Physiol Ther 2001;24(1):2–11.

[36] Pickar JG. Neurophysiological effects of spinal manipulation. Spine J 2002;2(5):357–371.

[37] Dishman JD, Bulbulian R. Spinal reflex attenuation associated with spinal manipulation. Spine 2000;25(19):2519–2524.

[38] Dishman JD, Ball KA, Burke J. First Prize: Central motor excitability changes after spinal manipulation: a transcranial magnetic stimulation study. J Manipulative Physiol Ther 2002;25(1):1–9.

[39] Brenner AK, Gill NW, Buscema CJ, et al. Improved activation of lumbar multifidus following spinal manipulation: a case report applying rehabilitative ultrasound imaging. J Orthop Sports Phys Ther 2007;37(10):613–619.

[40] Holding DH. Principles of training. London: Pergamon Press; 1965.

[41] Lee TD, Swanson LR, Hall AL. What is repeated in a repetition? Effects of practice conditions on motor skill acquisition. Phys Ther 1991;71(2):150–156.

[42] Rawlings EI, Rawlings IL, Chen CS, et al. The facilitating effects of mental rehearsal in the acquisition of rotary pursuit tracking. Psychonomic Sci 1972;26:71–73.

[43] Jacobson E. Electrophysiology of mental activity. Am J Psychol 1932;44:676–694.

[44] Allami N, Paulignan Y, Brovelli A, et al. Visuo-motor learning with combination of different rates of motor imagery and physical practice. Exp Brain Res 2008;184(1):105–113.

[45] Yue G, Cole KJ. Strength increases from the motor programme: comparison of training with maximal voluntary and imagined muscle contraction. J Neurophysiol 1992;67(5):1114–1123.

[46] Kelsey B. Effects of mental practice and physical practice upon muscular endurance. Res Quart 1961;32(99):47–54.

[47] Jeannerod M. Neural simulation of action: A unifying mechanism for motor cognition. Neuroimage 2001;14:S103–S109.

[48] Page SJ. Mental practice: a promising restorative technique in stroke rehabilitation. Top Stroke Rehabil 2001;8(3):54–63.

[49] Page SJ, Levine P, Leonard A. Mental practice in chronic stroke: results of a randomized, placebo-controlled trial. Stroke 2007; 38(4):1293–1297.

[50] Saxton JM, Clarkson PM, James R, et al. Neuromuscular dysfunction following eccentric exercise. Med Sci Sports Exerc 1995;27(8):1185–1193.

[51] Bonfim TR, Paccola CAJ, Barela JA. Proprioceptive and behavior impairments in individuals with anterior cruciate ligament reconstructed knees. Arch Phys Med Rehabil 2003;84(8):1217–1223.

[52] Lackner JR, DiZio P. Adaptation to Coriolis force perturbation of movement trajectory; role of proprioceptive and cutaneous somatosensory feedback. Adv Exp Med Biol 2002;508:69–78.

[53] Alter MJ. Science of flexibility. Champaign, IL: Human Kinetics; 1996.

[54] Bobath B. The application of physiological principles to stroke rehabilitation. Practitioner 1979;223:793–794.

[55] Young DE, Schmidt RA. Augmented kinematic feedback for motor learning. J Mot Behav 1992;24(3):261–273.

[56] Maxwell JP, Masters RS, Eves FF. From novice to no know-how: a longitudinal study of implicit motor learning. J Sports Sci 2000;18(2):111–120.

[57] Holding DH, Macrae AW. Guidance, restriction and knowledge of results. Ergonomics 1964;7:289–295.

[58] Dickinson J. The training of mobile balancing under a minimal visual cue situation. Ergonomics 1966;11:169–175.

[59] Winstein CJ, Pohl PS, Lewthwaite R. Effects of physical guidance and knowledge of results on motor learning: support for the guidance hypothesis. Res Quart Exerc Sport 1994;65(4):316–323.

[60] Weeks DL, Kordus RN. Relative frequency of knowledge of performance and motor skill learning. Res Quart Exerc Sport 1998;69(3):224–230.

[61] Sullivan KJ, Kantak SS, Burtner PA. Motor learning in children: feedback effects on skill acquisition. Phys Ther 2008; 88(6):720–732.

[62] Fitts PM, Posner MI. Human performance. Brooks/Cole; 1967.

[63] Adams JA. Short-term memory for motor responses. J Exp Psychol 1966;71(2):314–318.

[64] Koelbaek JM. Generalised muscular hyperalgesia in chronic whiplash syndrome. Pain 1999;83(2):229–234.

[65] French B, Thomas LH, Leathley MJ, et al. Repetitive task training for improving functional ability after stroke. Cochrane Database Syst Rev 2007;4: CD006073.

[66] Platz T, Bock S, Prass K. Behaviour among motor stroke patients with good clinical recovery: does it indicate reduced automaticity? Can it be improved by unilateral or bilateral training? A kinematic motion analysis study. Neuropsychologia 2001;39(7):687–698.

[67] Osgood CE. The similarity paradox in human learning: a resolution. Psychol Rev 1949;56:132–143.

[68] Heitkamp HC, Horstmann T, Mayer F, et al. Gain in strength and muscular balance after balance training. Int J Sports Med 2001;22(4):285–290.

[69] Asseman F, Caron O, Cremieux J. Is there a transfer of postural ability from specific to unspecific postures in elite gymnasts? Neurosci Lett 2004;358:83–86.

[70] Sale DG. Neural adaptation to resistance training. Med Sci Sports Exerc 1988;20:5.

[71] Dragana MC, Golubović J, Bratić M. Motor learning in sports. Phys Educ Sport 2004;2(1):45–59.

[72] Morris SL, Sharpe MH. PNF revisited. Physiother Theory Pract 1993;9:43–51.

[73] Cratty BJ. Movement behaviour and motor learning. 2nd ed. London: Henry Kimpton; 1967.

[74] Schlicht J, Camaione DN, Owen SV. Effect of intense strength training on standing balance, walking speed, and sit-to-stand performance in older adults. J Gerontol A Biol Sci Med Sci 2001;56(5):M281–M286.

[75] Sullivan KJ, Brown DA, Klassen T, et al. Effects of task-specific locomotor and strength training in adults who were ambulatory after stroke: results of the STEPS randomized clinical trial. Phys Ther 2007; 87(12):1580–1602 . discussion 1603–1607.

[76] Flansbjer UB, Miller M, Downham D, et al. Progressive resistance training after stroke: effects on muscle strength, muscle tone, gait performance and perceived participation. J Rehabil Med 2008;40 (1):42–48.

[77] Dean CM, Channon EF, Hall JM. Sitting training early after stroke improves sitting ability and quality and carries over to standing up but not to walking: a randomised trial. Aust J Physiother 2007;53(2):97–102.

[78] van de Port IG, Wood-Dauphinee S, Lindeman E, et al. Effects of exercise training programs on walking competency after stroke: a systematic review. Am J Phys Med Rehabil 2007;86(11):935–951.

[79] Bogey R, Hornby GT. Gait training strategies utilized in poststroke rehabilitation: are we really making a difference? Top Stroke Rehabil 2007;14(6):1–8.

[80] de Haart M, Geurts AC, Huidekoper SC, Fasotti L, van Limbeek J. Recovery of standing balance in postacute stroke patients: a rehabilitation cohort study. Arch Phys Med Rehabil 2004;85(6):886–895.

[81] Genthon N, Rougier P, Gissot AS, et al. Contribution of each lower limb to upright standing in stroke patients. Stroke 2008;39(6):1793–1799.

[82] Muehlbauer T, Panzer S, Shea CH. The transfer of movement sequences: effects of decreased and increased load. Q J Exp Psychol (Colchester) 2007;60(6):770–778.

[83] Wilde H, Shea CH. Proportional and nonproportional transfer of movement sequences. Q J Exp Psychol (Colchester) 2006;59(9):1626–1647.

[84] Dean NJ, Kovacs AJ, Shea CH. Transfer of movement sequences: bigger is better. Acta Psychol (Amst) 2008;127(2):355–368.

[85] Buchanan JJ, Zihlman K, Ryu YU, et al. Learning and transfer of a relative phase pattern and a joint amplitude ratio in a rhythmic multijoint arm movement. J Mot Behav 2007;39(1):49–67.

[86] LaFiandra M, Wagenaar RC, Holt KG, et al. How do load carriage and walking speed influence trunk coordination and stride parameters? J Biomech 2003;36(1):87–95.

[87] Wong AM, Lan C. Tai chi and balance control. Med Sport Sci 2008;52:115–123.

[88] Birbaumer N. Motor learning: passing a skill from one hand to the other. Curr Biol 2007;17(23): R1024–R1026.

[89] Halsband U, Lange RK. Motor learning in man: a review of functional and clinical studies. J Physiol Paris 2006;99 (4–6):414–424.

[90] Munn J, Herbert RD, Gandevia SC. Contralateral effects of unilateral resistance training: a meta-analysis. J Appl Physiol 2004;96(5):1861–1866.

[91] Perez MA, Tanaka S, Wise SP, Sadato N, et al. Neural substrates of intermanual transfer of a newly acquired motor skill. Curr Biol 2007;17(21):1896–1902.

[92] Smeulders MJ, Kreulen M, Hage JJ, et al. Motor control impairment of the contralateral wrist in patients with unilateral chronic wrist pain. Am J Phys Med Rehabil 2002; 81(3):177–181.

[93] Jerosch J, Thorwesten L. Proprioceptive abilities of patients with post–traumatic instability of the glenohumeral joint. Z Orthop Ihre Grenzgeb 1998;136(3):230–237.

[94] Roberts D, Friden T, Stomberg A, et al. Bilateral proprioceptive

defects in patients with a unilateral anterior cruciate ligament reconstruction: a comparison between patients and healthy individuals. J Orthop Res 2000;18(4):565–571.

[95] Maslovat D, Chua R, Lee TD, Franks IM. Contextual interference: single task versus multi-task learning. Motor Control 2004;8:213–233.

[96] Green DP, Whitehead J, Sugden DA. Practice variability and transfer of a racket skill. Percept Mot Skills 1995;81(3 Pt 2):1275–1281.

[97] Kerr R, Booth B. Specific and varied practice of motor skill. Percept Mot Skills 1978; 46(2):395–401.

[98] Brady F. Contextual interference: a meta-analytic study. Percept Mot Skills 2004;99(1): 116–126.

[99] Dick MB, Hsieh S, Dick-Muehlke C. The variability of practice hypothesis in motor learning: does it apply to Alzheimer's disease? Brain Cogn 2000;44(3):470–489.

[100] Dick MB, Hsieh S, Bricker J. Facilitating acquisition and transfer of a continuous motor task in healthy older adults and patients with Alzheimer's disease. Neuropsychology 2003;17(2):202–212.

[101] Lin CH, Sullivan KJ, Wu AD, et al. Effect of task practice order on motor skill learning in adults with Parkinson disease: a pilot study. Phys Ther 2007;87(9):1120–1131.

[102] Holm I, Fosdahl MA, Friis A, et al. Effect of neuromuscular training on proprioception, balance, muscle strength, and lower limb function in female team handball players. Clin J Sport Med 2004;14(2):88–94.

[103] Myklebust G, Engebretsen L, Braekken IH, et al. Prevention of anterior cruciate ligament injuries in female team handball players: a prospective intervention study over three seasons. Clin J Sport Med 2003;13(2):71–78.

[104] Risberg MA, Holm I, Myklebust G, et al. Neuromuscular training versus strength training during first 6 months after anterior cruciate ligament reconstruction: a randomized clinical trial. Phys Ther 2007;87(6):737–750.

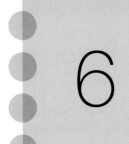

Plasticity in the motor system

Learning, retraining, motor reorganization in response to injury and return to functionality all imply that the motor system has the capacity to adapt to new experiences. Chapter 5 discussed the behavioural aspects of motor learning and how they can be used to promote sensory-motor adaptation. This chapter will examine the neurophysiological consequences of learning and their relevance to rehabilitation.

Sensory – motor adaptation

There are several neurophysiological processes associated with learning and sensory-motor adaptation (also termed *neural plasticity*).[1–3] They include changes in the neuronal cell surface and its filaments, sprouting of cell dendrites and axons, growth of new synaptic connections and changes in neurotransmitter release at the synapses. More recent studies have demonstrated neurogenesis (new neurons) within specific parts of the brain, in particular the hippocampus, an area associated with learning and memory. Neurogenesis has also been observed after brain damage in the areas of neural tissue repair.[4,5]

Plasticity in the motor system is not centre-specific but tends to occur within the whole sensory-motor system.[6] Tapping the index and middle finger of a monkey daily for several months was shown to change the cortical representation of the hand. The area representing the hand increased, distorting the cortical map in favour of the tapped fingers.[3] In blind Braille readers there is an expansion of the sensorimotor cortical representation of the reading finger.[7] Similarly in musicians, there is an increase in cortical representation of the playing fingers.[8] These changes in the cortex were shown to occur fairly rapidly, within 3 weeks of practising a novel task.[9] In the cerebellum, striatum and other motor-related cortical areas such changes are evident within a few days.[10] Interestingly, cortical reorganization is so rapid that it can even be demonstrated shortly after proprioceptive deprivation by an anesthetic block.[11]

Adaptive changes related to motor learning have been shown to take place even in the reflexive part of the motor system and spinal cord. Monkeys can be trained by the offer of a reward to depress or elevate the amplitude of the stretch reflex.[12–14] The reflex changes become evident within a few weeks to months and will persist for long periods of time, even after the removal of supraspinal influences, i.e. without the brain.[13] This implies that the spinal cord has the capacity to retain learned experiences. Humans can also be taught to control their stretch reflex, but it only takes nine practice sessions.[15] The reason for this difference may lie in the potent influence that cognition has in humans in accelerating the learning process (Ch. 5).

Further evidence for spinal cord "learning" was demonstrated in a study where animals that have only their spinal cord intact are trained to either stand or walk.[16] The results were task-specific learning where each group could only perform the task in which it was trained (walk or stand). Training each group in the other task reversed these two conditions, i.e. the walking group could be trained to stand, and vice versa. Once the activity was changed, the animal was unable to perform the previous motor task; a sort of competition in adaptation.

Central sensorimotor plasticity can also be demonstrated following injury in the periphery. In normal circumstances, the palm of the hand is used more than the dorsum and, therefore, the median nerve has a wider cortical representation. When the median nerve is cut, the cortical map of the hand will change in size in favour of the intact radial nerve. If the median nerve is allowed to regenerate, it will recapture some of its lost cortical territory.[17] Similarly, amputees or patients with spinal cord injuries show a lower threshold to excitation of muscles which are still innervated (proximal to the lesion).[18–20] This is attributed to enlarged sensorimotor representation of the unaffected proximal muscles and shrinkage of the sensorimotor representation of the denervated muscles.

Even less dramatic events such as immobilization and subsequently remobilization will result in motor adaptation.[21,22] It was demonstrated that during remobilization there was reorganization of the brain indicative of a "relearning" process.[23] Such plastic changes in response to immobilization can also be observed in the spinal motor centre.[24] Adaptive changes in the firing patterns of motor units can be demonstrated by straightforward joint immobilization.[25,26] Most of the adaptive changes took place within the first 3 weeks, probably beginning within days of immobilization.[23]

In patients with CNS damage the recovery of motor function is associated with motor reorganization in the brain.[27–32] Imaging studies have demonstrated that functional recovery of movement in the affected hand is brought about by the shift of neuronal recruitment to other areas of the brain; areas which previously were not involved in controlling that particular movement.

Peripheral plasticity – muscle, the acrobat of adaptation

By being a part of the neuromuscular continuum, muscle can exhibit dramatic adaptation in parallel to central plasticity.[33] Changes in the muscle can be in the form of length adaptation, hypertrophy and changes in the fibre type of the muscle.[34–43]

The adaptation in muscle tends to be fairly specific to the type of activity practised. Training in one form of activity, for example running, does not necessarily provide the neuromuscular adaptation required for, for example cycling (*specificity principle* in training), in the same way that the practice of yoga will not provide the adaptation required

for lifting weights. When learning a new movement pattern the muscle (and for that matter, the whole motor system) will readapt to the newly practised activity. In the muscle this involves a degree of fibre destruction (hence the delayed onset of muscle soreness) and adaptive reconstruction according to the new demands placed on it. Such adaptive changes in the muscle happen quite rapidly within 2–3 weeks.

The importance of physical challenges in adaptation

Physical challenges play an important role in promoting central reorganization and adaptation. In mice with partial spinal cord damage, treadmill training was shown to promote axonal sprouting and synapse formation proximal to the lesion and to improve motor recovery.[44] Even neurogenesis is driven by general physical activity or by providing challenging environments for the individual.[4,5]

However, not all exercises are equal. Motor learning that involves tasks such as coordination and balance encourages synaptogenesis, whereas treadmill exercise encourages the formation of new blood vessels in the brain (angiogenesis), with delayed synaptogenesis.[45–49] In a further study, synaptogenesis was evaluated using similar exercise protocols in animals with an induced stroke.[46,47] Synaptogenesis was evaluated after 14 and 28 days and was found to be intensively active within 14 days in the balance and coordination group, whereas in the treadmill group it was evident only at 24 days. Furthermore, in animals, early introduction of aerobic exercise after brain trauma tends to delay brain plasticity.[50,51] These studies have an important message for us:

Neuromuscular rehabilitation is not just about exercising. It is about providing cognitive-sensory-motor challenges that will facilitate motor learning/adaptation.

Hence, running on a treadmill could provide aerobic challenges and stimulate synaptogenesis (to a limit, otherwise marathon runners would have huge brains). However, running an obstacle course will be both aerobic and more cognitively demanding, since it involves more task variability and places greater challenges on various motor abilities. Similarly, playing a tennis game with a partner is more cognitively/motorically challenging than practising hitting a ball against a wall. These cognitive-motor challenges may, therefore, result in more complex sensory-motor reorganization. The message here is that rehabilitation should follow a similar strategy. It should provide challenges that vary, are cognitively demanding and are fun and interesting (depending on the patient's capacity). Avoid using "mindless" and tedious exercises.

Summary points

- Learning, retraining, motor organization to injury and return to functionality partly depend on the neurophysiological capacity of the motor system to adapt to new experiences.
- Motor adaptation is not centre-specific and can be observed throughout the neuromuscular continuum: brain, spinal cord and muscles.
- Central and peripheral adaptation occurs concurrently; separating them during treatment is artificial and ineffective. The muscle cannot be rehabilitated in isolation from its controller (the person).
- Rehabilitation is more about facilitating cognitive-sensory-motor processes and providing a stimulating and variations-rich environment. It is not just exercising.

References

[1] DeFeudis FV, DeFeudis PAF. Elements of the behavioral code. London: Academic Press; 1977.

[2] Rose S. The making of memory: from molecules to mind. London: Bantam Books; 1992.

[3] Kidd G, Lawes N, Musa I. Understanding neuromuscular plasticity: a basis for clinical rehabilitation. London: Edward Arnold; 1992.

[4] Kempermann G, van Praag H, Gage FH. Activity-dependent regulation of neuronal plasticity and self repair. Prog Brain Res 2000;127:35–48.

[5] Peterson DA. Stem cells in brain plasticity and repair. Curr Opin Pharmacol 2002;2(1):34–42.

[6] McComas AJ. Human neuromuscular adaptations that accompany changes in activity. Med Sci Sports Exerc 1994;26 (12):1498–1509.

[7] Pascual-Leone A, Cohen LG, Hallet M. Cortical map plasticity in humans. Trends Neurosci 1992;15(1):13–14.

[8] Elbert T, Pantev C, Wienbruch C, et al. Increased use of the left hand in string players associated with increased cortical representation of the fingers. Science 1995;220:21–23.

[9] Karni A, Meyer G, Rey-Hipolito C, et al. The acquisition of skilled motor performance: fast and slow experience-driven changes in primary motor cortex. Proc Nat Acad Sci USA 1998;95(3):861–868.

[10] Ungerleider LG, Doyon J, Karni A. Imaging brain plasticity during motor skill learning. Neurobiol Learn Mem 2002;78:553–564.

[11] Rossi S, Pasqualetti P, Tecchio F, et al. Modulation of corticospinal output to human hand muscles following deprivation of sensory feedback. Neuroimage 1998;8(2):163–175.

[12] Wolpaw JR. Adaptive plasticity in the spinal stretch reflex: an accessible substrate of memory? Cell Mol Neurobiol 1985; 5(1/2):147–165.

[13] Wolpaw JR, Carp JS, Lam Lee C. Memory traces in spinal cord produced by H-reflex conditioning: effects of post-tetanic potentiation. Neurosci Lett 1989a;103:113–119.

[14] Wolpaw JR, Lee CL. Memory traces in primate spinal cord produced by operant conditioning of H-reflex. J Neurobiology 1989;61(3):563–573.

[15] Evatt ML, Wolf SL, Segal RL. Modification of the human stretch reflex: preliminary studies. Neurosci Lett 1989;105:350–355.

[16] Hodgson JA, Roland RR, de-Leon R, et al. Can the mammalian lumbar spinal cord learn a motor task? Med Sci Sports Exerc 1994;26(12): 1491–1497.

[17] Wall JT, Kaas JH, Sur M, et al. Functional reorganization in somatosensory cortical areas 3b and 1 of adult monkeys after median nerve repair: possible relationships to sensory recovery in humans. J Neurosci 1986;6(1):218–233.

[18] Merzenich MM. Functional maps of skin sensations. In: Brown CC, editor. The many faces of touch, vol. 10. Pediatric Round Table Series. Johnson & Johnson Baby Products Company; 1984. p. 15–22.

[19] Cohen LG, Bandinelli S, Findley TW, et al. Motor reorganization after upper limb amputation in man. A study with focal magnetic stimulation. Brain 1991;114(1B):615–627.

[20] Elbert T, Sterr A, Flor H, et al. Input-increase and input-decrease types of cortical reorganization after upper extremity amputation in humans. Exp Brain Res 1997;117(1):161–164.

[21] Kaneko F, Murakami T, Onari K, et al. Decreased cortical excitability during motor imagery after disuse of an upper limb in humans. Clin Neurophysiol 2003;114(12):2397–2403.

[22] Liepert J, Tegenthoff M, Malin JP. Changes of cortical motor area size during immobilization. Electroencephalogr Clin Neurophysiol 1995;97:382–386.

[23] Seki K, Taniguchi Y, Narusawa M. Effects of joint immobilization on

firing rate modulation of human motor units. J Physiol 2001;530(3):507–519.

[24] Patten C, Kamen G. Adaptations in motor unit discharge activity with force control training in young and older human adults. Eur J Appl Physiol 2000; 83(2–3):128–143.

[25] Duchateau J, Hainaut K. Effects of immobilization on contractile properties, recruitment and firing rates of human motor units. J Physiol 1990;422:55–65.

[26] de Jong BM, Coert JH, Stenekes MW, et al. Cerebral reorganisation of human hand movement following dynamic immobilisation. Neuroreport 2003;14(13):1693–1696.

[27] Cramer SC, Nelles G, Benson RR, et al. A functional MRI study of subjects recovered from hemiparetic stroke. Stroke 1997;28:2518–2527.

[28] Cramer SC, Finklestein SP, Schaechter JD, et al. Activation of distinct motor cortex regions during ipsilateral and contralateral finger movements. J Neurophysiol 1999;81:383–387.

[29] Cao Y, D'Olhaberriague L, Vikingstad EM, et al. Pilot study of functional MRI to assess cerebral activation of motor function after poststroke hemiparesis. Stroke 1998;29(1):112–122.

[30] Brion JP, Demeurisse G, Capon A. Evidence of cortical reorganization in hemiparetic patients. Stroke 1989; 20(8):1079–1084.

[31] Rowe LB, Frackowiak RSJ. The impact of brain imaging technology on our understanding of motor function and dysfunction. Curr Opin Neurobiol 1999;9(6):728–734.

[32] Schaechter JD, Kraft E, Hilliard TS, et al. Motor recovery and cortical reorganization after constraint-induced movement therapy in stroke patients: a preliminary study. Neurorehabil Neural Repair 2002;16(4): 326–338.

[33] Henneman E. Skeletal muscle: the servant of the nervous system. In: Mountcastle VB, editor. Medical physiology. 4th ed. St Louis: Mosby; 1980. p. 674–702.

[34] Williams PE, Catanese T, Lucey EG, et al. The importance of stretch and contractile activity in the prevention of connective tissue accumulation in muscle. J Anat 1988;158:109–114.

[35] Singer B, Dunne J, Singer KP, et al. Evaluation of triceps surae muscle length and resistance to passive lengthening in patients with acquired brain injury. Clin Biomech (Bristol, Avon) 2002;17(2):152–161.

[36] Lehmann JF, Price R, deLateur BJ, et al. Spasticity: quantitative measurements as a basis for assessing effectiveness of therapeutic intervention. Arch Phys Med Rehabil 1989; 70(1):6–15.

[37] Gleim GW, McHugh MP. Flexibility and its effects on sports injury and performance. Sports Med 1997;24(5):289–299.

[38] Magnusson SP, Simonsen EB, Aagaard P, et al. A mechanism for altered flexibility in human skeletal muscle. J Physiol 1996;497(1):291–298.

[39] Bamman MM, Shipp JR, Jiang J, et al. Mechanical load increases muscle IGF-I and androgen receptor mRNA concentrations in humans. Am J Physiol, Endocrinol Metab 2001;280(3): E383–E390.

[40] Baldwin KM, Haddad F. Skeletal muscle plasticity: cellular and molecular responses to altered physical activity paradigms. Am J Phys Med Rehabil 2002;81(11 Suppl):S40–S51.

[41] McKoy G, Ashley W, Mander J, et al. Expression of insulin growth factor-1 splice variants and structural genes in rabbit skeletal muscle induced by stretch and stimulation. J Physiol 1999;516(Part 2):583–592.

[42] Yang H, Alnaqeeb M, Simpson H, et al. Changes in muscle fibre type, muscle mass and IGF-I gene expression in rabbit skeletal muscle subjected to stretch. J Anat 1997;190(Part 4): 613–622.

[43] Goldspink G. Changes in muscle mass and phenotype and the expression of autocrine and systemic growth factors by muscle in response to stretch and overload. J Anat 1999;194(Part 3):323–334.

[44] Goldshmit Y, Lythgo N, Galea MP, et al. Treadmill training after spinal cord hemisection in mice promotes axonal sprouting and synapse formation and improves motor recovery. J Neurotrauma 2008;25(5):449–465.

[45] Black JE, Isaacs KR, Anderson BJ, et al. Learning causes synaptogenesis, whereas motor activity causes angiogenesis, in cerebellar cortex of adult rats. Proc Nat Acad Sci USA 1990;87(14):5568–5572.

[46] Ding Q, Vaynman S, Akhavan M, et al. Insulin-like growth factor I interfaces with brain-derived neurotrophic factor-mediated synaptic plasticity to modulate aspects of exercise-induced cognitive function. Neuroscience 2006;140(3):823–833.

[47] Ding Y, Li J, Clark J, et al. Synaptic plasticity in thalamic nuclei enhanced by motor skill training in rat with transient middle cerebral artery occlusion. Neurolog Res 2003; 25(2): 189–194.

[48] Anderson BJ, Li X, Alcantara AA, et al. Glial hypertrophy is associated with synaptogenesis following motor-skill learning, but not with angiogenesis following exercise. Glia 1994;11(1):73–80.

[49] Anderson BJ, Alcantara AA, Greenough WT. Motor-skill learning: changes in synaptic organization of the rat cerebellar cortex. Neurobiol Learn Mem 1996;66(2):221–229.

[50] Griesbach GS, Gómez-Pinilla F, Hovda DA. The upregulation of plasticity-related proteins following TBI is disrupted with acute voluntary exercise. Brain Res 2004;1016(2):154–162.

[51] Griesbach GS, Gómez-Pinilla F, Hovda DA. Time window for voluntary exercise-induced increases in hippocampal neuroplasticity molecules after traumatic brain injury is severity dependent. J Neurotrauma 2007;24(7):1161–1171.

Motor reorganization in musculoskeletal injury

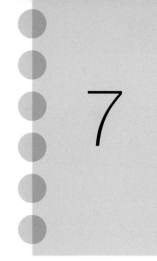

7

Musculoskeletal injury or pain will bring about profound cognitive, behavioural and motor control responses that serve to protect the body from further damage.[1,2] This response to injury is termed here *the injury response*.

In this chapter we will explore how the motor system reorganizes movement in injury and what influence it will have on the motor abilities. It will also discuss in which situations should neuromuscular rehabilitation be used and at what point after injury it should be introduced. The chapter will also examine the relationship between long-term motor reorganization and recurrent injury and progressive joint/tissue damage.

The injury response

There seems to be a "standard" motor response to damage or pain no matter which area or tissue is affected in the body. This injury response often manifests as a slowing down of movement, a loss of force, reduced movement range and an increase in fatigability. It is as if the motor system has used a "dimmer switch" to turn down the four movement parameters (force, velocity, length/range, endurance, Fig. 7.1). Furthermore, to ensure that the individual will not be tempted to physically stress their injury, within the psychological dimension, another inhibiting process kicks into action: the curbing of the "will to move". The individual will have an emotional experience of pain, fear of use, sense of weakness and loss of the will to carry out the movement.

This reorganization to injury can be put on hold during disastrous life-threatening events to allow the individual to reach safety. Hence, a person with a moderate leg or trunk injury may be able to escape from a burning house. Later, when there is perceived safety, the injury response will take over and in a matter of hours the person will become motorically unable to move. However, this injury response will be overrun by a survival response if this period of recuperation is suddenly interrupted by another life-threatening event. The person may find that they are, again, able to move using the injured limb.

There is an important point to this short story. The motor system can "switch" the injury response "off or on", depending on priorities. In musculoskeletal injury the motor system is healthy and well functioning compared to the tissues which are undergoing repair. There is no motor dysfunction, motor pathology or movement dysfunction here. This reorganization is a positive and well-orchestrated response.

In musculoskeletal injury the tissue damage is a set quantity at any point in time, e.g. the number of torn muscle fibres. On the other hand, the motor response is a variable entity. The magnitude of the whole response, or elements within it, can alter on a moment-to-moment basis depending on numerous factors. Apart from the severity of tissue damage, they include physiological needs (having to walk to find food), socio-economic realities (having to go to work with back pain) and psychological factors such as the "will" of the individual, health beliefs, mood, motivation, fear or depression. This

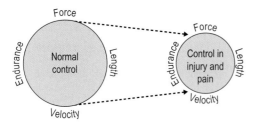

Fig. 7.1 • The "standard" injury response – a protection strategy which includes the turning down of the four movement parameters.

highlights the fact that the organization to movement is a complex multidimensional process and not a crude, stereotypic "stimulus-response" reflex (although there is some of this in it). It also means that motor control in injury can be more effectively rehabilitated by treatment that embraces the psychological/cognitive and behavioural dimensions of the individual (Ch. 8). These have potent and often dominant modulating influences over the more reflexive control elements.[3–7] For example, during movement subjects with high fear avoidance tend to reduce the force of their trunk muscles by half.[8–10] It implies that their force losses can be recovered by cognitive changes without any trunk-strengthening exercise!

It should be emphasised that the injury response can be initiated during any pain experience even in the absence of tissue damage or inflammation. The system may "mistake" the pain for being an injury. This is often observed in the non-traumatic and chronic pain conditions (Ch. 9).

The motor system in injury

In response to damage, information about the damage arrives to the central nervous system (CNS) from nociceptors and proprioceptors (Fig. 7.2). This information together with the cognitive/emotional experience of the injury will be integrated to organize for the injury. The next stage in this process is the selection and activation of the motor programme that will modify posture and movement in relation to the injury. It would be interesting to know whether these programmes for injury are learned responses or are pre-existing templates. It seems that we all immediately "know" what postures to adopt when injured (anyone for a PhD?).

Once the appropriate response has been selected the motor output will ensue, with the individual exhibiting the movement patterns associated with their injury.[11,12] It seems that there can be several responses to any one injury. Each individual uses their own unique movement patterns. Such variation between individuals has been observed in impingement syndrome of the shoulder and chronic neck pain conditions.[13,14] This has been also demonstrated in subjects with anterior cruciate deficient knees, where each person seems to have an individual compensating strategies during walking.[15] Furthermore, an injured person may demonstrate several "movement solutions" to a given task.

These injury responses are task-dependent and would, therefore, change between different activities.[16,17,18] It is also likely that the organization for injury changes over time.[19,20]

Fig. 7.2 • Motor organization for preventing further damage after injury.

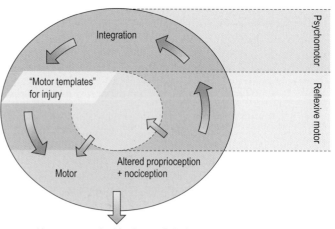

The signalling of damage

The signalling from the body is a mix of information about tissue damage from nociception and information from proprioception about the mechanical changes in the affected tissues.[21] The perception of pain is evoked by the information from nociceptors and other receptors, such as mechanoreceptors from the skin, muscles and joints, which also contribute to the sensation of pain.[22,23]

Proprioceptors can signal damage and promote motor reorganization in the absence of pain. When the knee is effused with non-painful saline it will initiate an inhibition of quadriceps motoneurons akin to the reflex patterns seen during knee injury.[24] Similarly, non-noxious stimulation of the glenohumeral joint capsule will elicit strong inhibition of the shoulder muscles (see arthrogenic inhibition below).[25]

Conscious awareness and the experience of injury will also have profound influence on the organization around injury. It may increase the levels of pain, increase movement incapacity and may even impede the rate of recovery.[6,16,26,27] Generally, injuries that are psychologically traumatic, such as road traffic accidents, are more likely to have such negative influences.[28,29]

The injury response and motor abilities

The turning down of the four movement parameters implies the involvement of the parametric and synergistic abilities in motor reorganization during injury (Fig. 7.3).[30]

It is expected that these abilities will be selective to the affected limb. However, local changes may be accompanied by complex whole-body pain/damage avoidance reorganization.[26] In patients with lower back pain (LBP) motor reorganization can be demonstrated even in the unaffected upper limb.[30] Furthermore, injuries affecting control on one side of the body may have a low-level cross-over to the opposite side.[31]

Composite abilities such as local coordination may also be affected.[26,32] They are expected to be associated with chronic musculoskeletal conditions, where movement dysfunction is progressing from an injury to a more chronic adaptive response. This is seen in situations where prolonged hand immobilization leads to local losses in coordination.[33] Another possibility is that composite abilities, such as postural stability/balance and coordination, may *appear* to have been affected.[34–36] However, they

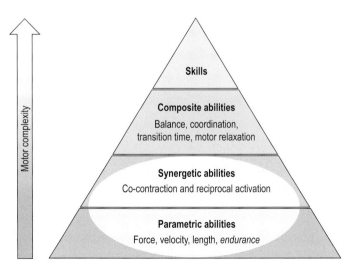

Fig. 7.3 • In the injury response the parametric abilities are affected within a synergistic level (change in one of the synergistic pairs is likely to affect the other in the pair). It will also have a knock-on effect on the composite abilities.

may represent the knock-on effects of changes in synergistic abilities and proprioception.

Force control

Patients with acute or chronic conditions will often complain of feeling that their joints or muscles are weak and that they fatigue easily.[37,38] This experience may sometime persist long after the pain has been alleviated and repair seems to be fully resolved.

There is a biological logic in this mechanism. Forceful muscle activation will raise the intramuscular as well as the intracapsular pressure and may result in further damage to these tissues.[61,62]

The force losses could be attributed to two processes. In the psychological dimension patients with musculoskeletal damage will be reluctant to fully activate their muscles because of fear of pain, and in the conscious sense there is a localized weakness and inability to successfully execute the movement.[7,39–41] This may lead to disuse atrophy, in particular if the patient is withdrawing from physical activities. In the neurological dimension, another more reflexive mechanism reduces the gain of the spinal motoneurons in response to joint damage. This is often called *arthrogenic inhibition* or *failure of voluntary activation* (Fig. 7.4). The outcome of this is more localized force loss, reduced endurance and, consequently, muscle wasting.[37,38]

Arthrogenic inhibition has been observed in acute knee effusion and inflammation,[42–48] in a chronically damaged knee (anterior cruciate ligament [ACL] tears, osteoarthritis [OA] of the knee and ageing) and in the elbow joint.[34–36,49–52] A similar process probably underlies the wasting of the multifidus and psoas muscles seen in patients with chronic lower back and neck pain.[53–59] Such muscle wasting can occur fairly rapidly. In acute lower back patients wasting of multifidus has been observed within 24 hours of pain onset.[55] Individuals who maintain physical activities after their injuries tend to reduce the negative effects of arthrogenic inhibition.[52,60]

Length control

Another strategy to prevent more damage is to limit the range of movement by muscle bracing.[63] The most dramatic demonstration of this is seen in acute conditions, such as acute torticolis or acute lower back pain, where the patient is immobilized rigidly

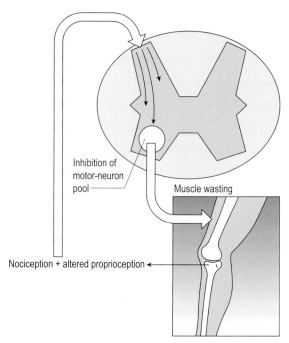

Fig. 7.4 • Arthrogenic inhibition in joints leading to muscle wasting.

by muscle contractions.[64,65] Probably this bracing strategy is achieved by an increase in localized co-contraction combined with hyper-reactive control to the muscles that restrict the movement towards damage.[64–67]

This controlled narrowing of range has also been observed in chronic conditions. In normal subjects during full forward bending the spinal extensor muscles tend to become inactive at the end range. However, in subjects with chronic back pain these muscles remain active even at the end range. Also in chronic back pain there is an increase in localized bracing by co-contraction, which will further limit the movement range.[7,68] These control elements are all part of a strategy that aims to keep the person upright and prevent them from bending – movements which would otherwise overload the damaged/painful posterior spinal structures.[7,69,70]

Such organization to limit the extent of movement can be seen also in painful muscle. When a muscle is injected with a painful irritant there is an inhibition of the painful muscle and excitation of muscles antagonistic to the movement.[71–73] Similarly, when pain is induced in tibialis anterior there is reduced joint movement in the limb during walking, which is controlled by a decrease in activity of the tibialis anterior and gastrocnemius muscles (synergistic control).[71]

Velocity control

Another hallmark of the injury response is slowness of movement.[11,12,63,74–76] Individuals with back pain reduce their walking speed and when pain is severe they seem to move almost as if in slow motion. Often the crucial indication that they are improving is that their movement speed begins to recover.

The slowing-down response is mediated within the psychological/psychomotor dimension affecting overall movement, as well as within the neurological dimension as a localized reflex response directed to muscles at the area of damage.[67,77]

Neuromuscular endurance

One way of reducing stresses on a damaged area is to prevent the person from repeatedly loading it by reducing endurance.[37,38] Localized, diminished neuromuscular endurance can be observed even in the absence of pain.[19,37,38,69,78–80]

Synergistic abilities

Co-contraction and reciprocal activation are profoundly affected following tissue damage and in pain conditions.[81] Several control factors can change in injury:

1. The relative force, velocity, muscle length between the synergistic pairs

2. Augmentation or diminution of one of the synergistic patterns

3. The *timing* and *duration* of activation between the synergists.

At synergistic level, the reorganization of the parametric abilities is represented as changes in the *relative* forces, velocities, lengths and fatigability between muscle pairs. Such reorganization can be observed in knee effusion where there may be force losses in the quadriceps coupled with an increase in hamstrings reactivity (Fig. 7.5).[47] Even fatigue or delayed muscle soreness in one muscle group will have an influence on control of the non-exercised synergists.[82–85]

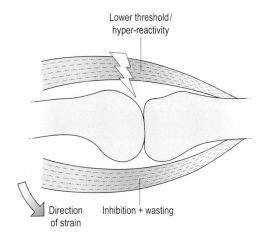

Lower threshold/hyper-reactivity

Direction of strain   Inhibition + wasting

Fig. 7.5 • Synergistic protective strategy to prevent further damage. Inhibition and weakness of muscle that pulls the joint into further strain and an increase in reactivity of the muscles that resist that movement.

A diminution of one of the synergistic patterns can be observed in different conditions. Functional instability is often the outcome of co-contraction inhibition.[49,86–90] In the ankle joint it often manifests as a sudden "giving way" during foot contact. This control failure seems to be sustained long after the tissues have recovered and may predispose the individual to recurrent ankle injury.[90]

An increase in the dominance of co-contraction strategy can be observed in lower back patients.[91] Co-contraction is considered to be an important control strategy to maintain spinal stability.[92,93] Patients suffering from low back pain tend to use higher levels of co-contraction force to increase stability, but also limit the range of movement (Fig. 7.6). They also have different reciprocal activation patterns of trunk muscles, indicative of synergistic

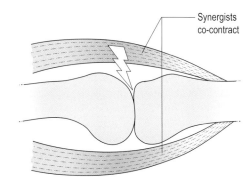

Synergists co-contract

Fig. 7.6 • Joint bracing is a synergistic co-contraction pattern to increase stability and reduce the movement range.

reorganization.[91,94–96] These control changes can be observed in every muscle group in the trunk, diaphragm and beyond.[91,97,98] Remember, even muscles that are inactive have a role within the synergistic control strategy (Ch. 2).

Changes in timing and duration

The timing of activation of synergistic muscle group during co-contraction and reciprocal activation are also affected in injury and pain. Everything is possible here: from changes in onset timing to changes in the duration of activation.[67,99] Delay in peroneal onset times can be observed in ankle and in tibialis anterior when this muscle is injected with an irritant.[90,100] Patients with anterior cruciate repair were shown to have longer onset times of hamstring muscles activation.[101] It is expected that all these timing differences would also affect the synergistic pair.

Synergistic timing can be very complex. This can be demonstrated in a study of trunk muscles activation during sudden trunk loading:

> . . .for healthy control subjects a shut-off of agonistic muscles (with a reaction time of 53 msec) occurred before the switch-on of antagonistic muscles (with a reaction time of 70 msec). Patients exhibited a pattern of co-contraction, with agonists remaining active (3.4 out of 6 muscles switched off) while antagonists switched on (5.3 out of 6 muscles). Patients also had longer muscle reaction times for muscles shutting off (70 msec) and switching on (83 msec) and furthermore, their individual muscle reaction times showed greater variability.[67]

This kind of complexity is not clinically friendly. It is not possible to test it or to even remember all of these minute details. Further complexity is introduced as this motor reorganization changes on a moment-to-moment basis during different postural and movement situations, i.e. these strategies are task-dependent. For example, during sudden postural challenges the onset timing of transverses abdominis can change depending on variables such as the phase of breathing,[98] different velocities and direction of arm movement,[102] and position of the trunk.[103] In chronic lower back patients these timings tend to be reorganized, but still remain complex task-dependent patterns (Ch. 2).[103–108]

Important clinical note

The fine motor changes described above are often single events within a more complex motor reorganization.[109] They represent a moment in time within a particular task carried out in the lab. It is very easy to lose track of the whole person/response and to be hooked on single control aspects such as timing of transversus abdominis or the cross-sectional area of multifidus at L4-5 in CLBP. They represent different aspects of a larger reorganization (see Table 3.1, Chapter 3) and, therefore, these single factors should not be the ultimate therapeutic goal.

How to resolve this problem of complexity is not to worry about it too much. It is virtually impossible to analyse injury organization muscle by muscle or reflex by reflex. Rehabilitation should ultimately focus on overall control. *Think movement not muscles!*

To treat or not to treat

It was put forward above that the injury response is a healthy motor control reorganization to prevent further injury. The question that arises is whether we can improve on this system and is there a time that we should intervene.

The immediate short-term reorganization of the neuromuscular system after injury should not be the focus of rehabilitation. This protective function often resolves when repair is complete and pain is alleviated (Fig. 7.7). If it didn't, we would all suffer from progressive motor disability from our multiple injuries throughout life. Perhaps in the first 2–3 weeks after injury the neuromuscular system should be left alone to do what it does best. All that is needed is for the patient to keep being active to facilitate this natural recovery, i.e. no specific rehabilitation is required. For example, we know that patients with acute lower back pain need no extra exercise to get better. The advice is to keep being active.[110,111] Generally, individuals who keep up with their physical activities after injury have less pain and a better motor control status than those who withdraw from activity.[19,60] However, overall management including gradual exposure, goal-setting, and cognitive-behavioural reassurance and empowerment can be helpful for some patients during the acute phase (Ch. 8).

So when does the injury response become dysfunctional? This occurs when the injury response is

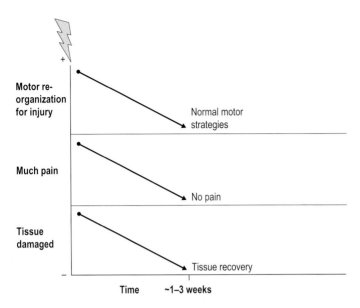

Fig. 7.7 • Acute injury. Motor re-organization serves a positive protective function.

maintained in the absence of a repair process, i.e. it serves no obvious functional/protective purpose and is impeding normal movement. There are four potential mechanisms that can account for maintaining a dysfunctional organization:

1. Severe injury or post-operative conditions where the repair is taking longer than usual to resolve (Fig. 7.8).[32] The injury response becomes the dominant movement strategy through the process of neuromuscular plasticity/adaptation. Consequently, the protective patterns may persist after tissue repair has been fully resolved.[112]

2. Physical constraints or immobilization that leads to a dysfunctional motor adaptation (Fig. 7.8). For example hand immobilization may lead to loss of coordination due to disuse (seen as plastic changes within the spinal cord and brain).[33]

3. Sensitization conditions where tissue damage has resolved but has remained painful (Fig. 7.9). Under these circumstances the CNS/individual may perceive pain as being an indication of damage and maintain a protective movement strategy, such as seen in individuals suffering from chronic lower back or neck pain.[113]

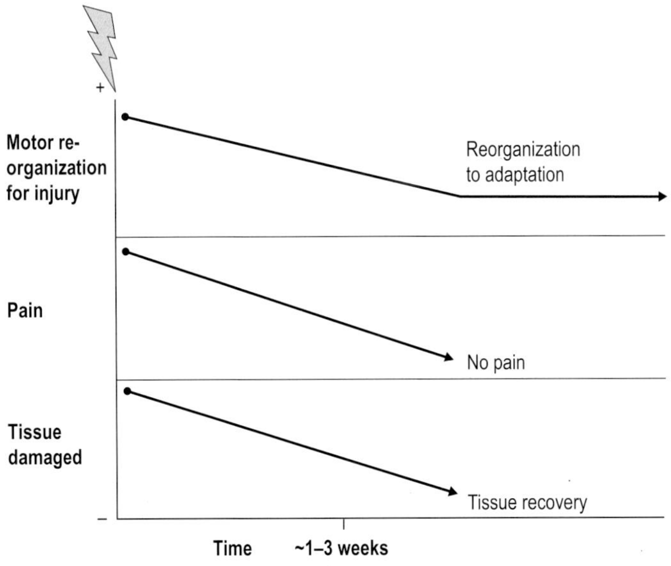

Fig. 7.8 • Sensitization conditions where tissue damage has resolved but has remained painful. Under these circumstances the central nervous system/individual may perceive pain as being an indication of damage and maintain a protective movement strategy.

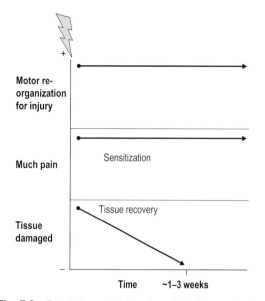

Fig. 7.9 • Physical constraints or immobilization may lead to a dysfunctional motor adaptation.

4. Psychological distress leading to "psychomotor" movement losses, such as seen in depression, anxiety conditions or high levels of fear-avoidance and catastrophizing (Fig. 7.10).[3–7]

The therapeutic intention may change for the different groups, but the rehabilitation is often very similar. In the group that is recovering from injury or is sensitized and where there is no obvious psychological distress (e.g. fear-avoidance), the intention is to help to recover motor losses. In patients where there is high psychological distress but low

evidence of tissue damage, rehabilitation is still the same, but the underlying therapeutic intention is to provide behavioural reassurance and empowerment, even in the absence of motor losses (Ch. 8).

Can the motor changes lead to further injury or progressive damage?

The short answer to this is we don't know. The evidence is mixed and not well-researched. In this model, altered control results in abnormal mechanical stresses being imposed on the joints/tissues. This is believed to lead to further damage or recurrent injury.[49,87,89,114–116] This is supported by some evidence that motor instability, such as seen in ankle sprains, can lead to future recurrences.[86,90,117,118] Also there is some evidence that athletes with sluggish reaction times are more prone to back and knee injuries.[119,120]

However, in a 20-year follow-up study of patients with chronic ankle instability, degenerative changes were observed only in six of 46 ankles, with no correlation to age or persistent instability.

There is also an interesting observation from working with stroke patients. It seems that the affected hand does not develop degenerative changes, although they suffer extensive motor control losses.[121] Similarly, ambulatory chronic stroke patients don't seem to develop any progressive joint or soft-tissue damage in the affected lower limb

Fig. 7.10 • Psychological distress may lead to "psychomotor" movement reorganization that resembles an injury response.

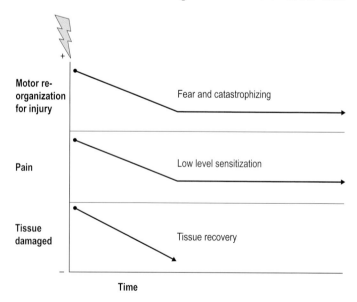

(unless they have an injury due to loss of control). But what is very surprising is how little these stroke patients suffer from back complaints, even though they have severe motor control losses to the trunk/spine.

As noted earlier, if motor losses led to progressive damage we would never recover from our injuries. We would forever be in a negative loop of injury leading to motor loss, to further injury, further motor loss and so on. Imagine even an uncomplicated injury such as the low level of damage associated with delayed-onset muscle soreness after exercise. Although it is associated with motor reorganization/losses,[122–124] most athletes will exercise during that period, seemingly without further progression of muscle damage.

Perhaps motor losses are more of an issue to individuals such as athletes who challenge their control of movement to the extremes of physical performance? But then we must suspect that all individuals have some motor losses related to past or current physical history and that these can be tolerated up to a certain point. Otherwise it would mean that athletes would be plagued with recurrent and progressive musculoskeletal pain and disability.

We need many more studies to establish how much control changes can be tolerated and how motor changes may interact with other factors to promote further damage.

Clinical note

The primary aim of neuromuscular rehabilitation is to help individuals to recover their control movement. It is unknown if rehabilitation would confer protective function against progressive tissue damage in the future.

Summary points

- The motor reorganization following injury is a multi-dimensional strategy culminating in postural and movement reorganization aimed at reducing the mechanical stresses imposed on the damaged tissues – in this text it is referred to as *the injury response.*

- The injury response is a positive healthy response and not a motor dysfunction or pathology.

- This response is highly individualistic. It is a dynamic process changing on a moment-to-moment basis during different phases of repair, levels of pain, re-injuries, underlying pathologies, ageing, and psychological states, such as anxiety, stress and depression.

- Acute musculoskeletal injuries should be left alone – the body know best.

- Neuromuscular rehabilitation is useful when the injury response serves no obvious protective function. It includes:

  ○ conditions where the injury response has become an adaptive state, such as in chronic recovery from injury or surgery or conditions where there were movement constraints or immobilization

  ○ sensitization conditions where tissue damage has resolved but has remained painful

  ○ injury-related psychological distress that leads to "psychomotor" movement losses.

- Parametric and synergistic motor abilities are the ones most likely to be affected in musculoskeletal injuries.

- Composite abilities may change as a knock-on effect from parametric and synergistic abilities.

- Don't get dazzled by scientific descriptions of the minute reflexive motor changes in injury – don't lose sight of the forest for the trees.

- *Think movement not muscles.*

References

[1] van Dieen JH, Selen LPJ, Cholewicki J. Trunk muscle activation in low-back pain patients, an analysis of the literature. J Electromyogr Kinesiol 2003;13(4):333–351.

[2] Schaible HG, Grubb BD. Afferents and spinal mechanisms of joint pain. Pain 1993;55:5–54.

[3] Adkin AL, Campbell AD, Chua R, Carpenter MG. The influence of postural threat on the cortical response to unpredictable and predictable postural perturbations. Neurosci Lett 2008;435(2):120–125.

[4] Lamoth CJ, Daffertshofer A, Meijer OG, Lorimer Moseley G, Wuisman PI, Beek PJ. Effects of experimentally induced pain and fear of pain on trunk coordination and back muscle activity during walking. Clin Biomech (Bristol, Avon) 2004;19(6):551–563.

[5] Lamoth CJ, Stins JF, Pont M, et al. Effects of attention on the control of locomotion in

individuals with chronic low back pain. J Neuroeng Rehabil 2008;5:13.

[6] Moseley GL, Hodges PW. Reduced variability of postural strategy prevents normalization of motor changes induced by back pain: a risk factor for chronic trouble? Behav Neurosci 2006;120(2):474–476.

[7] Cholewicki J, van Dieen JH, Arsenault AB. Muscle function and dysfunction in the spine. J Electromyogr Kinesiol 2003;13(4):303–304.

[8] Thomas JS, France CR, Lavender SA, et al. Effects of fear of movement on spine velocity and acceleration after recovery from low back pain. Spine 2008;33(5):564–570.

[9] Thomas JS, France CR, Sha D, et al. The influence of pain-related fear on peak muscle activity and force generation during maximal isometric trunk exertions. Spine 2008;33(11):E342–E348.

[10] Thomas JS, France CR. Pain-related fear is associated with avoidance of spinal motion during recovery from low back pain. Spine 2007;32(16):E460–E466.

[11] Lamoth CJ, Daffertshofer A, Meijer OG, et al. How do persons with chronic low back pain speed up and slow down? Trunk-pelvis coordination and lumbar erector spinae activity during gait. Gait Posture 2006;23(2):230–239.

[12] Lamoth CJ, Meijer OG, Daffertshofer A, et al. Effects of chronic low back pain on trunk coordination and back muscle activity during walking: changes in motor control. Eur Spine J 2006;15(1):23–40.

[13] Roy JS, Moffet H, McFadyen BJ. Upper limb motor strategies in persons with and without shoulder impingement syndrome across different speeds of movement. Clin Biomech (Bristol, Avon) 2008;23(10):1227–1236. Epub 2008 Aug 30.

[14] Sjölander P, Michaelson P, Jaric S, et al. Sensorimotor disturbances in chronic neck pain – range of motion, peak velocity, smoothness of movement, and repositioning acuity. Man Ther 2008;13(2):122–131.

[15] Torry MR, Decker MJ, Ellis HB, et al. Mechanisms of compensating for anterior cruciate ligament deficiency during gait. Med Sci Sports Exerc 2004;36(8):1403–1412.

[16] Moseley GL, Nicholas MK, Hodges PW. Does anticipation of back pain predispose to back trouble? Brain 2004;127(Part 10):2339–2347.

[17] Falla D, Farina D, Dahl MK, Graven-Nielsen T. Muscle pain induces task-dependent changes in cervical agonist/antagonist activity. J Appl Physiol. 2007; 102(2):601–609.

[18] Thomas JS, France CR, Sha D, et al. The effect of chronic low back pain on trunk muscle activations in target reaching movements with various loads. Spine 2007;32(26):E801–E808.

[19] Bandholm T, Rasmussen L, Aagaard P, et al. Force steadiness, muscle activity, and maximal muscle strength in subjects with subacromial impingement syndrome. Muscle Nerve 2006; 34(5):631–639.

[20] Bandholm T, Rasmussen L, Aagaard P, et al. Effects of experimental muscle pain on shoulder-abduction force steadiness and muscle activity in healthy subjects. Eur J Appl Physiol 2008;102(6):643–650.

[21] Falla D, Farina D, Graven-Nielsen T. Experimental muscle pain results in reorganization of coordination among trapezius muscle subdivisions during repetitive shoulder flexion. Exp Brain Res 2007;178(3):385–393.

[22] Casey KL. Neural mechanisms of pain. In: Carterette EC, Friedman MP, editors. Handbook of perception: feeling and hurting. London: Academic Press; Ch 6, 1978. p. 183–219.

[23] Meyer RA, Campbell JA, Raja S. Peripheral neural mechanisms of nociception. In: Wall PD, Melzack R, editors. Textbook of pain. 3rd ed. London: Churchill Livingstone; 1994. p. 13–42.

[24] Wood L, Ferrell WR, Baxendale RH. Pressures in normal and acutely distended human knee joints and effects on quadriceps maximal voluntary contractions. Q J Exp Physiol 1988;73:305–314.

[25] Voigt M, Jakobsen J, Sinkjaer T. Non-noxious stimulation of the glenohumeral joint capsule elicits strong inhibition of active shoulder muscles in conscious human subjects. Neurosci Lett 1998;254:105–108.

[26] Arendt–Nielsen L, Graven–Nielsen T, Svarrer H, et al. The influence of low back pain on muscle activity and coordination during gait: a clinical and experimental study. Pain 1996; 64(2):231–240.

[27] Buitenhuis J, de Jong PJ, Jaspers JP, et al. Relationship between posttraumatic stress disorder symptoms and the course of whiplash complaints. J Psychosom Res 2006;61(5): 681–689.

[28] Nederhand MJ, Hermens HJ, Ijzerman MJ, Groothuis KG, Turk DC. The effect of fear of movement on muscle activation in posttraumatic neck pain disability. Clin J Pain 2006; 22(6):519–525.

[29] Graven-Nielsen T, Arendt-Nielsen L. Impact of clinical and experimental pain on muscle strength and activity. Curr Rheumatol Rep 2008;10(6): 475–481.

[30] Leinonen V, Airaksinen M, Taimela S, et al. Low back pain suppresses preparatory and triggered upper-limb activation after sudden upper-limb loading. Spine 2007;32(5):E150–E155.

[31] Hortobagyi T, Taylor JL, Petersen NT, et al. Changes in segmental and motor cortical output with contralateral muscle contractions and altered sensory inputs in humans. J Neurophysiol 2003;90(4):2451–2459.

[32] van Uden CJ, Bloo JK, Kooloos JG, et al. Coordination and stability of one-legged hopping patterns in patients with anterior cruciate ligament reconstruction: preliminary results. Clin Biomech 2003; 18(1):84–87.

[33] de Jong BM, Coert JH, Stenekes MW, et al. Cerebral reorganisation of human hand movement following dynamic

immobilisation. Neuroreport 2003;14(13):1693–1696.

[34] Hurley MV, Scott DL, Rees J, et al. Sensorimotor changes and functional performance in patients with knee osteoarthritis. Ann Rheum Dis 1997;56(11): 641–648.

[35] Hurley MV, Rees J, Newham DJ. Quadriceps function, proprioceptive acuity and functional performance in healthy young, middle-aged and elderly subjects. Age Ageing 1998; 27(1):55–62.

[36] Hassan BS, Mockett S, Doherty M. Static postural sway, proprioception, and maximal voluntary quadriceps contraction in patients with knee osteoarthritis and normal control subjects. Ann Rheum Dis 2001;60(6):612–618.

[37] Roy SH, De Luca CJ, Casavant DA. Lumbar muscle fatigue and chronic lower back pain. Spine 1989;14(9): 992–1001.

[38] Taimela S, Kankaanpaa M, Luoto S. The effect of lumbar fatigue on the ability to sense a change in lumbar position. A controlled study. Spine 1999; 24(13):1322–1327.

[39] Rainville J, Ahern DK, Phalen L, et al. The association of pain with physical activities in chronic low back pain. Spine 1992;17(9): 1060–1064.

[40] Verbunt JA, Seelen HA, Vlaeyen JW, et al. Disuse and deconditioning in chronic low back pain: concepts and hypotheses on contributing mechanisms. Eur J Pain 2003; 7(1):9–21.

[41] Verbunt JA, Seelen HA, Vlaeyen JW, et al. Fear of injury and physical deconditioning in patients with chronic low back pain. Arch Phys Med Rehabil 2003;84(8):1227–1232.

[42] Spencer JD, Hayes KC, Alexander IJ. Knee joint effusion and quadriceps reflex inhibition in man. Arch Phys Med Rehabil 1984;65:171–177.

[43] Stokes M, Young A. The contribution of reflex inhibition to arthrogenous muscle weakness. Clin Sci 1984;67:7–14.

[44] Iles JF, Stokes M, Young A. Reflex actions of knee joint afferents during contraction of the human quadriceps. Clin Physiol 1990;10:489–500.

[45] Jones DW, Jones DA, Newham DJ. Chronic knee effusion and aspiration: the effect on quadriceps inhibition. Br J Rheumatol 1987;26:370–374.

[46] Kennedy JC, Alexander IJ, Hayes KC. Nerve supply of the human knee and its functional importance. Am J Sports Med 1982;10(6):329–335.

[47] Torry MR, Decker MJ, Viola RW, et al. Intra-articular knee joint effusion induces quadriceps avoidance gait patterns. Clin Biomech 2000;15(3):147–159.

[48] Sharma L. Proprioceptive impairment in knee osteoarthritis. Rheum Dis Clin North Am 1999;25(2):299–314.

[49] Hurley MV, Newham DJ. The influence of arthrogenous muscle inhibition on quadriceps rehabilitation of patients with early, unilateral osteoarthritic knees. Br J Rheumatol 1993;32:127–131.

[50] Fisher NM, Pendergast DR. Reduced muscle function in patients with osteoarthritis. Scand J Rehabil Med 1997;29(4): 213–221.

[51] Chmielewski TL, Stackhouse S, Axe MJ, et al. A prospective analysis of incidence and severity of quadriceps inhibition in a consecutive sample of 100 patients with complete acute anterior cruciate ligament rupture. J Orthop Res 2004;22(5):925–930.

[52] Hurley MV, O'Flanagan DJ, Newham SJ. Isokinetic and isometric muscle strength and inhibition after elbow arthroplasty. J Orthop Rheumatol 1991;4:83–95.

[53] Takemasa R, Yamamoto H, Tani T. Trunk muscle strength in and effect of trunk muscle exercises for patients with chronic low back pain. The differences in patients with and without organic lumbar lesions. Spine 1995;20(23):2522–2530.

[54] Hides JA, Richardson CA, Jull GA. Multifidus muscle recovery is not automatic after resolution of acute, first-episode low-back-pain. Spine 1996;21:2763–2769.

[55] Hides JA, Stokes MJ, Saide M, et al. Evidence of lumbar multifidus muscle wasting ipsilateral to symptoms in patients with acute/subacute low back pain. Spine 1994;19:165–172.

[56] Danneels LA, Vanderstraeten GG, Cambier DC, et al. CT imaging of trunk muscles in chronic low back pain patients and healthy control subjects. Eur Spine J 2000;9(4): 266–272.

[57] Cooper RG, St Clair Forbes W, Jayson MI. Radiographic demonstration of paraspinal muscle wasting in patients with chronic low back pain. Br J Rheumatol 1992;31(6):389–394.

[58] Fernández-de-las-Peñas C, Albert-Sanchís JC, Buil M, et al. Cross-sectional area of cervical multifidus muscle in females with chronic bilateral neck pain compared to controls. J Orthop Sports Phys Ther 2008;38(4):175–180.

[59] Wallwork TL, Stanton WR, Freke M, et al. The effect of chronic low back pain on size and contraction of the lumbar multifidus muscle. Man Ther 2008; Epub 2008 Nov 20.

[60] Solomonow M, Baratta R, Zhou BH, et al. The synergistic action of the anterior cruciate ligament and thigh muscles in maintaining joint stability. Am J Sports Med 1987;15(3): 207–213.

[61] Racinais S, Bringard A, Puchaux K, Noakes TD, Perrey S. Modulation in voluntary neural drive in relation to muscle soreness. Eur J Appl Physiol 2008;102(4):439–446.

[62] Alexander C, Caughey D, Withy S, et al. Relation between flexion angle and intraarticular pressure during active and passive movement of the normal knee. J Rheumatol 1996;23 (5):889–895.

[63] Moseley GL, Hodges PW. Are the changes in postural control associated with low back pain caused by pain interference? Clin J Pain 2005;21(4):323–329.

[64] Holm S, Indahl A, Solomonow M. Sensorimotor

control of the spine.
J Electromyogr Kinesiol 2002;
12(3):219–234.

[65] Solomonow M, Zhou BH, Harris M, et al. The ligamento-muscular stabilizing system of the spine. Spine 1998;23(23): 2552–2562.

[66] Solomonow M, Baratta RV, Zhou BH, et al. Muscular dysfunction elicited by creep of lumbar viscoelastic tissue. J Electromyogr Kinesiol 2003; 13(4):381–396.

[67] Zedka M, Prochazka A, Knight B, et al. Voluntary and reflex control of human back muscles during induced pain. J Physiol 1999;520 (Part 2):591–604.

[68] Marras WS, Ferguson SA, Burr D, Davis KG, Gupta P. Functional impairment as a predictor of spine loading. Spine 2005;30(7): 729–737.

[69] Shirado O, Ito T, Kaneda K, Strax TE. Flexion-relaxation phenomenon in the back muscles. A comparative study between healthy subjects and patients with chronic low back pain. Am J Phys Med Rehabil 1995;74(2):139–144.

[70] Kaigle AM, Wessberg P, Hansson TH. Muscular and kinematic behavior of the lumbar spine during flexion-extension. J Spinal Disord 1998;(11):163–174.

[71] Graven-Nielsen T, Svensson P, Arendt-Nielsen L. Effects of experimental muscle pain on muscle activity and co-ordination during static and dynamic motor function. Electroencephalogr Clin Neurophysiol/Electromyogr Motor Control 1997;105(2):156–164.

[72] Svensson P, Miles TS, McKay D, et al. Suppression of motor evoked potentials in a hand muscle following prolonged painful stimulation. Eur J Pain 2003;7(1):55–62.

[73] Farina D, Arendt-Nielsen L, Merletti R, et al. The effect of experimental muscle pain on motor unit firing rate and conduction velocity. J Neurophysiol 2004;91:1250–1259.

[74] Manetta J, Franz LH, Moon C, et al. Comparison of hip and knee muscle moments in subjects with and without knee pain. Gait Posture 2002;16(3):249–254.

[75] Lindsay D, Horton J. Comparison of spine motion in elite golfers with and without low back pain. J Sports Sci 2002;20(8):599–605.

[76] Coulthard P, Pleuvry BJ, Brewster M, et al. Gait analysis as an objective measure in a chronic pain model. J Neurosci Meth 2002;116(2):197–213.

[77] Luoto S, Taimela S, Hurri H, et al. Psychomotor speed and postural control in chronic low back pain patients. A controlled follow-up study. Spine 1996; 21(22):2621–2627.

[78] Kumbhare DA. Measurement of cervical flexor endurance following whiplash. Disabil Rehabil 22; 2005;27(14):801–807.

[79] Suter E, Lindsay D. Back muscle fatigability is associated with knee extensor inhibition in subjects with low back pain. Spine 2001;26(16):E361–E366.

[80] Shirado O, Ito T, Kaneda K, et al. Concentric and eccentric strength of trunk muscles: influence of test postures on strength and characteristics of patients with chronic low-back pain. Arch Phys Med Rehabil 1995;76(7):604–611.

[81] Fu SN, Hui-Chan CW. Modulation of prelanding lower-limb muscle responses in athletes with multiple ankle sprains. Med Sci Sports Exerc 2007;39(10): 1774–1783.

[82] Weir JP, Keefe DA, Eaton JF, et al. Effect of fatigue on hamstring coactivation during isokinetic knee extensions. Eur J Appl Physiol Occup Physiol 1998;78(6):555–559.

[83] Maynard J, Ebben WP. The effects of antagonist prefatigue on agonist torque and electromyography. J Strength Cond Res 2003;17(3):469–474.

[84] Semmler JG, Tucker KJ, Allen TJ, et al. Eccentric exercise increases EMG amplitude and force fluctuations during submaximal contractions of elbow flexor muscles. J Appl Physiol 2007;103(3):979–989.

[85] Nyland JA, Caborn DN, Shapiro R. Fatigue after eccentric quadriceps femoris work produces earlier gastrocnemius and delayed quadriceps femoris activation during crossover cutting among

normal athletic women. Knee Surg Sports Traumatol Arthrosc 1997; 5(3):162–167.

[86] Freeman MAR, Dean MRE, Hanham IWF. The etiology and prevention of functional instability of the foot. J Bone Joint Surg (B) 1965;47(4):678–685.

[87] Skinner HB, Barrack RL, Cook SD, Haddad Jr RJ. Joint position sense in total knee arthroplasty. J Orthop Res 1984;1:276–283.

[88] Cratty BJ. Movement behaviour and motor learning. 2nd ed. London: Henry Kimpton; 1967.

[89] Barrack RL, Skinner HB, Cook SD, et al. Effect of articular disease and total knee arthroplasty on knee joint-position sense. J Neurophysiol 1983;50(3):684–687.

[90] Richie Jr DH. Functional instability of the ankle and the role of neuromuscular control: a comprehensive review. J Foot Ankle Surg 2001;40(4):240–251.

[91] Danneels LA, Coorevits PL, Cools AM, et al. Differences in electromyographic activity in the multifidus muscle and the iliocostalis lumborum between healthy subjects and patients with sub-acute and chronic low back pain. Eur Spine J 2002;11 (1):13–19.

[92] Manohar M, Panjabi MM. Clinical spinal instability and low back pain. J Electromyogr Kinesiol 2003;13(4):371–379.

[93] Stokes IA, Gardner-Morse M. Spinal stiffness increases with axial load: another stabilizing consequence of muscle action. J Electromyogr Kinesiol 2003; 13(4):397–402.

[94] Hubley-Kozey CL, Vezina MJ. Differentiating temporal electromyographic waveforms between those with chronic low back pain and healthy controls. Clin Biomech 2002;17 (9–10): 621–629.

[95] Hemborg B, Moritz U. Intra-abdominal pressure and trunk muscle activity during lifting. II. Chronic low-back patients. Scand J Rehabil Med 1985;17(1):5–13.

[96] Radebold A, Cholewicki J, Polzhofer GK, et al. Impaired postural control of the lumbar

spine is associated with delayed muscle response times in patients with chronic idiopathic low back pain. Spine 2001;26(7):724–730.

[97] Leinonen V, Kankaanpää M, Airaksinen O, Hänninen O. Back and hip extensor activities during trunk flexion/extension: effects of low back pain and rehabilitation. Arch Phys Med Rehabil 2000;81(1):32–37.

[98] Hodges PW, Butler JE, McKenzie DK, Gandevia SC. Contraction of the human diaphragm during rapid postural adjustments. J Physiol 1997; 505(Part 2):539–548.

[99] Leinonen V, Kankaanpaa M, Luukkonen M, et al. Disc herniation-related back pain impairs feed-forward control of paraspinal muscles. Spine 2001;26(16):E367–E372.

[100] Madeleine P, Voigt M, Arendt-Nielsen L. Reorganisation of human step initiation during acute experimental muscle pain. Gait Posture 1999;10(3):240–247.

[101] Bonfim TR, Jansen Paccola CA, Barela JA. Proprioceptive and behavior impairments in individuals with anterior cruciate ligament reconstructed knees. Arch Phys Med Rehabil 2003;84:1217 1223.

[102] Hodges PW, Richardson CA. Relationship between limb movement speed and associated contraction of the trunk muscles. Ergonomics 1997b; 40(11):1220–1230.

[103] Hodges PW, Richardson CA. Delayed postural contraction of transversus abdominis in low back pain associated with movement of the lower limb. J Spinal Disord 1998;11(1):46–56.

[104] Hodges PW, Richardson CA. Inefficient muscular stabilization of the lumbar spine associated with low back pain. A motor control evaluation of transversus abdominis. Spine 1996;21(22): 2640–2650.

[105] Hodges PW, Richardson C. Altered trunk muscle recruitment in people with low back pain with upper limb movement at different speeds. Arch Phys Med Rehabil 1999; 80(9):1005–1012.

[106] Hodges PW, Gandevia SC, Richardson CA. Contractions of specific abdominal muscles in postural tasks are affected by respiratory maneuvers. J Appl Physiol 1997;83(3):753–760.

[107] Hodges PW, Richardson CA. Delayed postural contraction of transversus abdominis in low back pain associated with movement of the lower limb. J Spinal Disord 1998;11(1): 46–56.

[108] Hodges PW, Moseley GL, Gabrielsson A, et al. Experimental muscle pain changes feedforward postural responses of the trunk muscles. Exp Brain Res 2003;151(2): 262–271.

[109] Asay JL, Mündermann A, Andriacchi TP. Adaptive patterns of movement during stair climbing in patients with knee osteoarthritis. J Orthop Res 2008;27(3):325–329.

[110] Liddle SD, Gracey JH, Baxter GD. Advice for the management of low back pain: a systematic review of randomised controlled trials. Man Ther 2007;12(4):310–327.

[111] Hagen KB, Hilde G, Jamtvedt G, et al. Bed rest for acute low back pain and sciatica. Cochrane Database Syst Rev 2004;(4): CD001254.

[112] Smith AJ, Lloyd DG, Wood DJ. Pre-surgery knee joint loading patterns during walking predict the presence and severity of anterior knee pain after total knee arthroplasty. J Orthop Res 2004;22(2):260–266.

[113] Koelbaek-Johansen M. Generalised muscular hyperalgesia in chronic whiplash syndrome. Pain 1999;83(2): 229–234.

[114] Palmieri-Smith RM, Kreinbrink J, Ashton-Miller JA, et al. Quadriceps inhibition induced by an experimental knee joint effusion affects knee joint mechanics during a single-legged drop landing. Am J Sports Med 2007;35(8):1269–1275.

[115] Parkhurst TM, Burnett CN. Injury and proprioception in the lower back. J Orthop Sports Phys Ther 1994;19(5):282–295.

[116] Zazulak B, Cholewicki J, Reeves NP. Neuromuscular control of trunk stability: clinical implications for sports injury prevention. J Am Acad Orthop Surg 2008;16(9):497–505.

[117] McVey ED, Palmieri RM, Docherty CL, et al. Arthrogenic muscle inhibition in the leg muscles of subjects exhibiting functional ankle instability. Foot Ankle Int 2005;26(12): 1055–1061.

[118] van Cingel RE, Kleinrensink G, Uitterlinden EJ, et al. Repeated ankle sprains and delayed neuromuscular response: acceleration time parameters. J Orthop Sports Phys Ther 2006;36(2):72–79.

[119] Cholewicki J, Silfies SP, Riaz RA, Shah A, et al. Delayed trunk muscle reflex responses increase the risk of low back injuries. Spine 2005;30(23): 2614–2620.

[120] Zazulak BT, Hewett TE, Reeves NP. Deficits in neuromuscular control of the trunk predict knee injury risk: a prospective biomechanical-epidemiologic study. Am J Sports Med 2007;35(7): 1123–1130.

[121] Segal R, Avrahami E, Lebdinski E, et al. The impact of hemiparalysis on the expression of osteoarthritis. Arthritis Rheum 1998;41(12): 2249–2256.

[122] Bottas R, Nicol C, Komi PV, et al. Adaptive changes in motor control of rhythmic movement after maximal eccentric actions. J Electromyogr Kinesiol 2007;19 (2):347–356. Epub 2007 Oct 15.

[123] Nie H, Arendt-Nielsen L, Kawczynski A, et al. Gender effects on trapezius surface EMG during delayed onset muscle soreness due to eccentric shoulder exercise. J Electromyogr Kinesiol 2007;17(4):401–409. Epub 2006 Jun 27.

[124] Bulbulian R, Bowles DK. Effect of downhill running on motoneuron pool excitability. J Appl Physiol 1992;73(3): 968–973.

Cognitive and behavioural considerations in neuromuscular rehabilitation

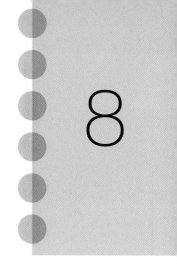

Cognitions, behaviours and movement control are profoundly interlaced and inseparable and should be considered as an essential part of patient care in neuromuscular rehabilitation (Fig. 8.1).

A person's beliefs, their attitudes and the action they take when they are injured or in pain can have important implications for their recovery. Furthermore, the individual's movement repertoire may contain particular habitual patterns that could put them at risk of injury. These beliefs and behaviour can be challenged in ways that could help the patient to adopt different attitudes and modify certain elements in their behaviour, changes that could facilitate recovery and reduce the potential for future injury.

Injury cognitions and behaviours

A patient who used to be a keen runner withdrew from this activity due to mild lower back pain. He was advised by his surgeon to stop jogging because it would exacerbate the wear and tear in his back. Another patient had knee pain as a consequence of a fall in judo. He believed that "knees can be a problem" and considered stopping judo. A 65-year-old tennis player had surgery of his serving shoulder. He had all the possible shoulder conditions known to humankind affecting this joint. Will he ever be able to play tennis again?

All these patients are exhibiting certain beliefs about their condition that hold them back from resuming these activities. These beliefs often manifest as *fear-avoidance* ("I can't walk because it

causes my back pain and it will make it worse") or *catastrophizing* ("I will never be able to walk again, I have to stop working.").[1-4] This group of patients is adapting their behaviour in response to pain, discomfort or movement losses, frequently withdrawing from activities that may help them to recover. Often these beliefs in combination with psychological and social factors predate the injury and could impact the potential for recovery. For example, the development of serious back pain disability can be predicted more accurately from psychosocial factors than from structural/degenerative changes in the spine.[5] The individual's beliefs about their condition may also be influenced by previous negative injury/surgery experiences.

As the injury/pain lingers on, these factors feed the widening discrepancy between the "real" physical losses and the patient's perceived inability (Fig. 8.2). For some individuals there is no such gap. They may suffer significant movement losses and may feel that their body has let them down.

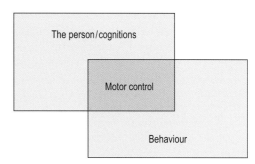

Fig. 8.1 • Cognitions, behaviours and movement control are profoundly interlaced and inseparable.

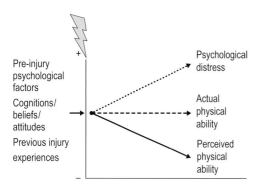

Fig. 8.2 • The patient's psychological distress about their injury may widen the gap between the actual and perceived physical ability. Their behaviour during the injury is often dictated by the perceived ability. Pre-injury factors such as psychosocial traits, health beliefs and attitudes, and previous experiences of injury/pain can influence their recovery.

Patients suffering from physical losses and ongoing painful conditions will often experience feelings such as disappointment, anger, frustration, grief, helplessness, loss of control and depression. Frequently, the individual will become more focused on their loss and dominated by their disability. Their identity is that of an injured self, experiencing a negative change in their body and self-image.[6–8] As time passes these psychological distresses may become more entrenched, further influencing the way the individual interacts with their environment.[9]

These psychological factors are as important as the physical aspect of the treatment and, therefore, should be addressed during rehabilitation.

Cognitions, beliefs and attitudes

Within the professional–ethical boundaries of manual and physical therapists there are several ways in which we can help our patients to transform their cognitions about their condition. This can manifest clinically as challenging their beliefs about the condition, focusing on positive attitudes and engaging their positive coping strategies. Our management will also aim to help the patient to contain their fears, anxieties and catastrophic thoughts by reassurance as well as by empowering them to self-care.[10–13] The outcome from such transformations can be reduced pain, improved movement ability, a return to more normal occupational and recreational activities, and less health-seeking behaviour.[10–17]

Cognition and behaviour are inseparable. Hence, change in cognitions such as fear-avoidance will influence the person's behaviour. Equally, challenging behaviour through the introduction of safe and non-aggravating movement experiences can influence how a person perceives their condition (Fig. 8.3).

There are several ways in which to assist the patient to transform their cognitions. Providing the patient with relevant information about their condition can be part of this process.[15,18,19] People who have a better understanding of their condition can be empowered to self-care more effectively and are more likely to initiate behavioural actions that challenge their fears. If we take one of the above examples, the patient with the knee condition, it was explained to him that his knee had got better within normal expected times (2–3 weeks), that the fact that he had no history of knee injury, and that such an injury does not cause osteoarthritis. This was enough to reassure him to return to judo (see also: Working with cognitions: changing the narrative, Ch. 9).

Also focusing on the "abled-self" rather than "disabled-self" can help to reassure, pointing out to the patient what they can do, rather than what they can't do. For example, I often see in clinic patients suffering from chronic back pain who are virtually symptom-free during demanding physical activities such as gardening, playing football or even windsurfing. The focus here would be on these "abled" activities – focusing on success. This approach also has a clinical manifestation. Movement rehabilitation often starts with what the patient is able to do and later experiments with their inability – start with the possible and then tease the impossible.

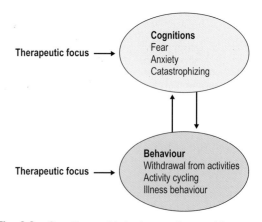

Fig. 8.3 • Cognition and behaviour are inseparable. Changes in cognition will influence behaviour and vice versa.

Further to the focus on the cognitive aspects, we must keep in mind the quality of the therapeutic relationship.[18] Clinical attitudes that include being attentive to the patient's emotional state, empathic, non-judgemental, caring and encouraging, will all have important implications for their process of recovery.[20]

Reassurance by actions: the behavioural experiment

Generally, after an injury most individuals will return to pre-injury activities in a gradual manner. They take a series of chances in which positive movement experiences embolden them to take further steps to improve the condition. However, there are some injuries where the actions a person takes result in pain and may lead to a gradual withdrawal from these activities – sometimes beyond what is required to prevent further damage. In this scenario there is a growing discrepancy between the magnitude of tissue damage and the person's perception of their injury and, therefore, their behaviour.

One therapeutic aim is to help the patient to narrow the discrepancy between the real and perceived losses. This can be achieved by implementing what most injured individuals do naturally: gradual exposure to the task. A graded challenge is a step-wise increase in a particular activity (Fig. 8.4). This grading can be achieved by increasing the duration, repetition or intensity of the remedial activity over time (think of expanding the four movement parameters – force, length, velocity and endurance).

A gradual challenge can have several clinical manifestations. It can start in the session during examination, where the patient is guided in movement patterns which they fear. For example, a patient with non-specific chronic lower back pain may be invited to perform different trunk movements or even jump gently on the spot. For those with long-term pain, and who are particularly apprehensive, the physical reassurance may start on the treatment table, as a challenge to the trunk in different movement patterns (see DVD section on trunk rehabilitation). All these physical challenges are carried out in a graded manner, within pain-free ranges and physically possible tasks and with the support and reassurance of the therapist.

Beyond the session the behavioural reassurance is to gradually expose the patient to the very movement and tasks which they fear.[11,12,21–23] The patient makes a wish-list of the exercise or activities in order of importance. If the exercise, say, is to return to tennis after a back injury, this would be set as one of the therapeutic goals. The graded challenge can start with serving a tennis ball against a wall for 5 minutes a day, gradually increasing the duration, intensity and number of serves over several weeks and so on.

It is important to involve the patient in the decision-making about the form of challenges, the scheduling of the exposure and the setting of short- and long-term goals.[24] Goal-setting is all about working out with the patient targets that are specific, measurable, attainable, relevant and have a realistic time scale (acronym SMART).

Behavioural reassurance can have a profound influence on recovery and should not be underestimated. It was demonstrated that in chronic back conditions, pain levels and functionality can improve equally well with cognitive-behavioural approaches as with physical exercise.[17,25] It seems that both approaches share similar underlying process for improvement – empowering and reassuring by reducing the levels of anxiety/fear/catastrophizing. The exercise training is a form of behavioural approach that challenges and helps to transform the individual's beliefs about their condition and attitudes to their body ("my back can do all this, so it must be OK"). The improvements observed in patient suffering from back pain have been attributed to these cognitive-behavioural factors rather than to the physical changes in trunk associated with exercising.[26]

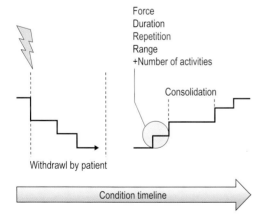

Force
Duration
Repetition
Range
+Number of activities

Consolidation

Withdrawl by patient

Condition timeline

Fig. 8.4 • The behavioural experiment includes a gradual increase of challenges in specific activities. The challenge is increased in a stepwise manner, widening the four movement parameters. At particular times it may be necessary to consolidate the improvements if the next step up aggravates the condition.

Behaviour and musculoskeletal pain

Some musculoskeletal injuries are just bad luck. However, many are acquired and to a certain extent preventable. Such injuries can be due to the way a person uses their body or the frequency or duration in performing specific tasks or movement patterns. These conditions seem to stem from within different spheres of behaviour, each requiring a unique form of management.

For this purpose behaviour can be categorized into several spheres (Fig. 8.5). There are behaviours that are associated with the interface between the person and their physical environment: the way a person bends to lift, holds a tennis racket and serves, walking patterns and so on. This will be termed here as *task-behaviour*. There is also the behaviour associated with the organization, sequencing and scheduling of tasks and routines. For example, how often the person is

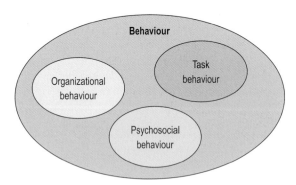

Fig. 8.5 • Spheres of behaviour. *Task-behaviour* is associated with the interface between the person and their physical environment. *Organizational-behaviour* is the behaviour associated with the organization, sequencing and scheduling of tasks and routines. *Psychosocial-behaviour* is associated with the relationships of the individual to others.

bending to lift, how often they are having breaks and so on. This will be termed here as *organizational-behaviour*. Another sphere of behaviour is associated with the relationships of the individual to others, which will be termed here *psychosocial-behaviour*. Acquiring musculoskeletal pain conditions or injuries can be associated with actions within any one of, or a combination of, these behavioural spheres.

Task-behaviour sphere

A person may develop musculoskeletal pain conditions or injury by the way they use their body in relation to their physical environment (task-behaviour).[11,12,22,27–33] For example, chronic neck pain can develop in individuals who spend many hours with their neck flexed in positions above 20 degrees.[31,32,34,35] Similarly, individuals who spend more than half a day sitting in an awkward position may develop lower back pain.[36] Individuals who are in an occupation that involves repetitive heavy lifting may have a slightly raised incidence of lower back pain.[37] In sports, certain landing techniques can result in knee injury.[38] In cyclists, an unsuitable seat height or bicycle position, or improperly adjusted pedal systems, may cause various lower-limb conditions.[39]

Within the task-behaviour sphere the aim of guidance is to improve the human–physical environment interface by either modifying behaviour itself or the environment. In the case of neck pain it might be to provide postural advice on ideal neck position or to make sure the computer screen is placed at a correct height, etc.[40,41] For the cyclist, it would be readjusting the bicycle to better suit the rider.[39]

Organizational-behaviour sphere

Sometimes injuries are related to the organizational sphere of behaviour (sequencing, scheduling and organization of a task). In this scenario a condition may be prevented or helped by a change in the scheduling and by introducing variations in the tasks. For example work-related lower back pain is associated with repetitive heavy lifting and prolonged standing.[37,42] Moderate positive improvements can be achieved in the organizational-behaviour sphere by encouraging the individual to return to work early and to ask to be given light duties and breaks, and by applying gradual exposure.[37] However, educating workers in bending and lifting techniques (task-behaviour) does not reduce the incidence of back pain/injury.[43] It seems that this condition is acquired within the organizational rather than the task-behaviour sphere.

In sport, changes introduced within the organizational-behaviour sphere may help to reduce the potential for injury. Some sports injuries are due to overuse and burnout or may be due to fatigue during competition/games[39,44,45] For example, runners and other endurance athletes can develop a wide range of overuse injuries in the lower limbs.[39] The management of this group of individuals should be within the organizational-behaviour sphere, by introducing breaks/rest periods to reduce fatigue/exhaustion during training and games.[39,45–49] On the other hand, guidance in the task-behaviour sphere, say, focusing on kicking or running technique, may be an ineffective intervention since the condition is acquired within a different sphere of behaviour.

Management in the organizational sphere is important for patients with chronic conditions who may find themselves in a negative loop – doing too much when they feel well, so being in more pain, then having to withdraw from physical activities, to be followed by a period of doing too much to catch up with time lost during withdrawal, and so on (termed *activity cycling*, Fig. 8.6). This can happen also to the "overdoers", often athletes, who exercise to the point of failure. This group of patients may benefit from a programme that combines gradual exposure and periods of rest (termed *pacing*).

Sometimes the management has to involve both task- and organizational-behaviour. For example, patients with work-related neck pain may benefit from postural advice (task-behaviour) as well as advice on breaks and coping with high work demands (organizational-behaviour).[40]

Psychosocial behaviour

In the last two decades it has become more evident that the progression of many conditions from acute to chronic state can be predicted by psychosocial factors such as low job satisfaction, low support at work, socio-economic background and psychological distress.[37,42,50,51]

The psychosocial-behavioural sphere is probably outside the scope of rehabilitation in manual and physical therapies. Where such factors are evident in the case history, the patient should be referred to professionals who specialize in this area of work.

Management in behavioural spheres: an example

A recent population study has demonstrated that work-related neck and upper limb pain is associated with repeated lifting of heavy objects, prolonged bending of the neck, and working with arms at/above shoulder height, little job control and little supervisor support.[52] Of this pain, 24% was attributed to exposure to work activities and 12% to exposure to psychosocial factors. Let's examine each of these factors and explore what the intervention might be:

1. Repeated lifting of heavy objects – unlikely to be able to change this work posture. Therefore, intervention is in the organizational-behaviour sphere. Solution: provide more frequent breaks, provide light duties or mixed tasks.

2. Prolonged bending of neck – task- and organizational-behaviour spheres. Solution: at the task-behaviour sphere, correct working posture including modifying the work station. On the organization-behavioural sphere, provide more frequent breaks and mix with alternative tasks.

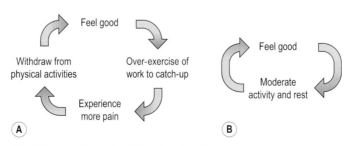

Fig. 8.6 • Activity cycling (A) and pacing (B).

3. Working with arms at/above shoulder height – as in 1.

4. Little job control and little supervisor support – this is occurring within the psychosocial-behavioural sphere and is, therefore, likely to be outside the management speciality of physical therapists.

Prevention of injury: more exercise or task-behaviour?

In regards to prevention of sports injury, several studies have demonstrated that the frequency of leg injuries can be reduced by adding a neuromuscular approach to training (a sort of functional exercising).[53–60] The aim of these approaches is to modify motor control of specific joints and to improve the position of, and minimize the stress on, specific joints. They are usually a mix of two rehabilitation approaches: one focused on underlying motor abilities by introducing functional tasks, and one focused on extra-functional challenges such as running, jumping, hopping and cutting tasks. The training also consists of movement education that emphasizes proper landing and cutting techniques (management in the task-behaviour sphere). This includes advice to land on the forefoot and roll back to the rear foot, to engage knee and hip in flexion and, where possible, to land on two feet. Players are trained to avoid excessive dynamic valgus of the knee and to focus on the "knee over toe position" when cutting.[38]

It is possible that movement education (task-behaviour) is the more important element in these training approaches rather than modifying motor control. The leg injuries often occur in healthy non-injured athletes and are, therefore, unlikely to be due to underlying motor control losses. Furthermore, the subjects are highly trained athletes who are already at peak motor performance. Many of the additional neuromuscular exercises emulate what the athletes do anyway in their sport and are, therefore, unlikely to add to their movement control during the game.

Summary points

- Cognition, behaviour and movement control are inseparable.
- Behaviour is the observable action of the individual.
- Certain beliefs, attitudes and behaviour can lead to chronicity that will affect movement control.
- Helping individuals to modify their injury behaviour and challenging their beliefs and attitudes about their condition can facilitate recovery.
- Musculoskeletal pain and injury can arise in normal individuals from habitual physically stressful or inefficient movement patterns, i.e. behaviour leading to injury or pain.
- Some injuries and pain conditions can be acquired by the way the person uses their body in relation to the physical environment (task-behaviour).
- Some injuries and pain conditions can be acquired by the way the person organizes and schedules their physical activities (organizational-behaviour).
- Helping individuals to modify their task and organizational-behaviour could help to prevent musculoskeletal injury and pain.
- Neuromuscular rehabilitation is not just about exercising.
- Movement control and behaviour can change solely by cognitive means.

References

[1] Poiraudeau S, Rannou F, Baron G, et al. Fear-avoidance beliefs about back pain in patients with subacute low back pain. Pain 2006;124:305–311.

[2] Leeuw M, Goossens ME, Linton SJ, Crombez G, Boersma K, Vlaeyen JW. The fear-avoidance model of musculoskeletal pain: current state of scientific evidence. J Behav Med 2007;30(1):77–94.

[3] Shaw WS, Pransky G, Patterson W, Linton SJ, Winters T. Patient clusters in acute, work-related back pain based on patterns of disability risk factors. J Occup Environ Med 2007;49(2): 185–193.

[4] Elfving B, Andersson T, Grooten WJ. Low levels of physical activity in back pain patients are associated with high levels of fear-avoidance beliefs and pain catastrophizing. Physiother Res Int 2007; 12(1):14–24.

[5] Carragee E, Alamin TF, Miller JL, Carragee JM. Discographic, MRI and psychosocial determinants of low back pain disability and remission: a prospective study in subjects with benign persistent back pain. Spine J 2005; 5(1):24–35.

[6] Moseley GL, Zalucki NM, Wiech K. Tactile discrimination, but not tactile stimulation alone, reduces chronic limb pain. Pain 2008a;137(3):600–608. Epub 2007 Dec 3.

[7] Moseley GL. I can't find it! Distorted body image and tactile dysfunction in patients with chronic back pain. Pain 2008b;140(1):239–243. Epub 2008 Sep 10.

[8] Lotze M, Moseley GL. Role of distorted body image in pain. Curr Rheumatol Rep 2007; 9(6):488–496. Review.

[9] Boersma K, Linton SJ. How does persistent pain develop? An analysis of the relationship between psychological variables, pain and function across stages of chronicity. Behav Res Ther 2005;43(11):1495–1507.

[10] Linton SJ, Ryberg M. A cognitive-behavioral group intervention as prevention for persistent neck and back pain in a non-patient population: a randomized controlled trial. Pain 2001; 90(1–2):83–90.

[11] Linton SJ, Boersma K, Jansson M, Svärd L, Botvalde M. The effects of cognitive-behavioral and physical therapy preventive interventions on pain-related sick leave: a randomized controlled trial. Clin J Pain 2005;21(2): 109–119.

[12] Linton SJ, Nordin E. A 5-year follow-up evaluation of the health and economic consequences of an early cognitive behavioral intervention for back pain: a randomized, controlled trial. Spine 2006;31(8):853–858.

[13] Williams AC, Richardson PH, Nicholas MK, et al. Inpatient vs. outpatient pain management: results of a randomised controlled trial. Pain 1996;66(1):13–22.

[14] Skinner JB, Erskine A, Pearce S, Rubenstein I, Taylor M, Foster C. The evaluation of a cognitive behavioural treatment programme in outpatients with chronic pain. J Psychosom Res 1990;34(1):13–19.

[15] Burton AK, Waddell G, Tillotson KM, et al. Information and advice to patients with back pain can have a positive effect.

A randomised controlled trial of a novel educational booklet in primary care. Spine 1999;24:2484–2491.

[16] Hoffman BM, Papas RK, Chatkoff DK, Kerns RD. Meta-analysis of psychological interventions for chronic low back pain. Health Psychol 2007;26(1): 1–9.

[17] Smeets RJ, Vlaeyen JW, Kester AD, et al. Reduction of pain catastrophizing mediates the outcome of both physical and cognitive-behavioral treatment in chronic low back pain. J Pain 2006;7(4):261–271.

[18] Linton SJ, Andersson T. Can chronic disability be prevented? A randomized trial of a cognitive-behavior intervention and two forms of information for patients with spinal pain. Spine 2000;25(21): 2825–2831.

[19] Moseley GL, Nicholas MK, Hodges PW. A randomized controlled trial of intensive neurophysiology education in chronic low back pain. Clin J Pain 2004;20(5):324–330.

[20] Lederman T. Touch as a therapeutic intervention. In: Liam T, editor. Morphodynamics of osteopathy. Germany: Hippokrates Verlag; 2006.

[21] Linton SJ. Occupational psychological factors increase the risk for back pain: a systematic review. J Occup Rehabil 2001; 11(1):53–66.

[22] Linton SJ, Boersma K, Jansson M, Overmeer T, Lindblom K, Vlaeyen JW. A randomized controlled trial of exposure in vivo for patients with spinal pain reporting fear of work-related activities. Eur J Pain 2008;12(6):722–730.

[23] Vlaeyen JWS, de Jong J, Geilen M, Heuts PH, van Breukelen G. The treatment of fear of movement/(re)injury in chronic low back pain: further evidence on the effectiveness of exposure in vivo. Clin J Pain 2002;18:251–261.

[24] Pfingsten M. Functional restoration – it depends on an adequate mixture of treatment. Schmerz 2001;15(6):492–498.

[25] Critchley DJ, Ratcliffe J, Noonan S, et al. Effectiveness and cost-effectiveness of three types of physiotherapy used to reduce chronic low back pain disability: a pragmatic randomized trial with economic evaluation. Spine 2007;32(14):1474–1478.

[26] Mannion AF, Muntener M, Taimela S, et al. A randomized clinical trial of three active therapies for chronic low back pain. Spine 1999;24:2435–2448.

[27] Gonge H, Jensen LD, Bonde JP. Do psychosocial strain and physical exertion predict onset of low-back pain among nursing aides? Scand J Work, Environ Health 2001;27(6):388–394.

[28] Watson KD, Papageorgiou AC, Jones GT, et al. Low back pain in schoolchildren: the role of mechanical and psychosocial factors. Arch Dis Child 2003; 88(1):12–17.

[29] Perez CE. Chronic back problems among workers. Health Reports/ Statistics Canada 2000; (1):41–55.

[30] Veiersted KB, Westgaard RH, Andersen P. Electromyographic evaluation of muscular work pattern as a predictor of trapezius myalgia. Scand J Work, Environ Health 1993;19(4):284–290.

[31] Ariens GA, van Mechelen W, Bongers PM, et al. Physical risk factors for neck pain. Scand J Work, Environ Health 2000; 26(1):7–19.

[32] Ariens GA, Bongers PM, Hoogendoorn WE, et al. High physical and psychosocial load at work and sickness absence due to neck pain. Scand J Work, Environ Health 2002;28(4):222–231.

[33] Hoogendoorn WE, Bongers PM, de Vet HC, et al. High physical work load and low job satisfaction increase the risk of sickness absence due to low back pain: results of a prospective cohort study. Occ Environ Health Med 2003;59(5):323–328.

[34] De Loose V, Burnotte F, Cagnie B, Stevens V, Van Tiggelen D. Prevalence and risk factors of neck pain in military office workers. Mil Med 2008;173(5):474–479.

[35] Cagnie B, Danneels L, Van Tiggelen D, De Loose V, Cambier D. Individual and work related risk factors for neck pain among office workers: a cross sectional study. Eur Spine J 2007;16(5):679–686.

[36] Lis AM, Black KM, Korn H, Nordin M. Association between sitting and occupational LBP. Eur Spine J 2006;16(2):283–298 . Epub 2006 May 31.

[37] Waddell G, Burton AK. Occupational health guidelines for the management of low back pain at work: evidence review. Occup Med 2001;51(2):124–135.

[38] Renstrom P, Ljungqvist A, Arendt E, et al. Non-contact ACL injuries in female athletes: an International Olympic Committee current concepts statement. Br J Sports Med 2008;42(6):394–412.

[39] Cosca DD, Navazio F. A series of medical interventions may effectively treat overuse injuries in adult endurance athletes. Am Fam Physician 2007;76:237–244.

[40] Bernaards CM, Ariëns GA, Knol DL, et al. The effectiveness of a work style intervention and a lifestyle physical activity intervention on the recovery from neck and upper limb symptoms in computer workers. Pain 2007; 132(1–2):142–153.

[41] Bernaards CM, Ariëns GA, Simons M, et al. Improving work style behavior in computer workers with neck and upper limb symptoms. J Occup Rehabil 2008;18(1):87–101.

[42] Andersen JH, Haahr JP, Frost P. Risk factors for more severe regional musculoskeletal symptoms: a two-year prospective study of a general working population. Arthritis Rheum 2007;56(4):1355–1364.

[43] Hartvigsen J, Lauritzen S, Lings S, et al. Intensive education combined with low tech ergonomic intervention does not prevent low back pain in nurses. Occup Environ Med 2005; 62(1):13–17.

[44] Perkins RH, Davis D. Musculoskeletal injuries in tennis. Phys Med Rehabil Clin N Am 2006;17(3):609–631.

[45] Cresswell SL, Eklund RC. Changes in athlete burnout over a thirty-week "rugby year" J Sci Med Sport 2006;9:125–134.

[46] Borotikar BS, Newcomer R, Koppes R, et al. Combined effects of fatigue and decision making on female lower limb landing postures: central and peripheral contributions to ACL injury risk. Clin Biomech (Bristol, Avon) 2008;23 (1):81–92.

[47] McLean SG, Felin RE, Suedekum N, et al. Impact of fatigue on gender-based high-risk landing strategies. Med Sci Sports Exerc 2007;39(3): 502–514.

[48] Kernozek TW, Torry MR, Iwasaki M. Gender differences in lower extremity landing mechanics caused by neuromuscular fatigue. Am J Sports Med 2008;36(3):554–565.

[49] Chappell JD, Herman DC, Knight BS, et al. Effect of fatigue on knee kinetics and kinematics in stop-jump tasks. Am J Sports Med 2005;33(7):1022–1029.

[50] Brage S, Sandanger I, Nygård JF. Emotional distress as a predictor for low back disability: a prospective 12-year population-based study. Spine 2007; 32(2):269–274.

[51] Bigos SJ, Battié MC, Spengler DM, et al. A prospective study of work perceptions and psychosocial factors affecting the report of back injury. Spine 1991;16(1):1–6.

[52] Sim J, Lacey RJ, Lewis M. The impact of workplace risk factors on the occurrence of neck and upper limb pain: a general population study. BMC Public Health 2006;6:234.

[53] Myklebust G, Engebretsen L, Braekken IH, et al. Prevention of anterior cruciate ligament injuries in female team handball players: a

prospective intervention study over three seasons. Clin J Sport Med 2003;13(2):71–78.

[54] Holm I, Fosdahl MA, Friis A, et al. Effect of neuromuscular training on proprioception, balance, muscle strength, and lower limb function in female team handball players. Clin J Sport Med 2004;14(2): 88–94.

[55] Petersen W, Zantop T, Steensen M, et al. Prevention of lower extremity injuries in handball: initial results of the handball injuries prevention programme. Sportverletz Sportschaden 2002;16(3): 122–126.

[56] Petersen W, Braun C, Bock W, et al. A controlled prospective case control study of a prevention training program in female team handball players: the German experience. Arch Orthop Trauma Surg 2005;125(9):614–621.

[57] Gilchrist J, Mandelbaum BR, Melancon H, et al. A randomized controlled trial to prevent noncontact anterior cruciate ligament injury in female collegiate soccer players. Am J Sports Med 2008;36(8): 1476–1483.

[58] Mandelbaum BR, Silvers HJ, Watanabe DS, et al. Effectiveness of a neuromuscular and proprioceptive training program in preventing anterior cruciate ligament injuries in female athletes: 2-year follow-up. Am J Sports Med 2005; 33(7):1003–1010.

[59] Hewett TE, Ford KR, Myer GD. Anterior cruciate ligament injuries in female athletes: Part 2, a meta-analysis of neuromuscular interventions aimed at injury prevention. Am J Sports Med 2006;34(3):490–498.

[60] Myer GD, Ford KR, Palumbo JP, et al. Neuromuscular training improves performance and lower-extremity biomechanics in female athletes. J Strength Cond Res 2005;19(1):51–60.

Managing non-traumatic pain conditions

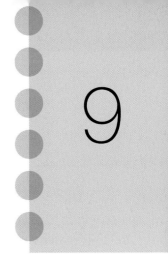

While writing this chapter, I was treating a 40-year-old patient for severe neck pain and stiffness which have developed over a period of 9 years. The patient had to stop driving because she was no longer able to turn her head. She had no history of neck trauma and the neck imaging was normal. Although active movements of her neck were severely restricted, the passive range was almost full, with pain only at the extreme ranges of rotation. Her condition started shortly after starting a new computer-based job, in which she experienced high levels of psychological stress. This case represents a large group of the patients who suffer from chronic (and acute) neck and shoulder pain conditions without any history of trauma.

There are several such acquired non-traumatic conditions that are now well documented. The upper body and arms seem to be common areas for these conditions, including chronic neck and shoulder pain, trapezius myalgia,[1–11] muscular jaw pain[12–25] and tension headaches.[26–30] Probably some of the chronic, non-specific back pains fall into the same group of conditions.

Although in different areas, it seems that many of these conditions share similar underlying processes.[22,24,31] They are all associated with psychological-behavioural factors, and are believed to be transmitted via the motor system to various muscles, which may, eventually, become painful (Fig. 9.1).

Traditionally these conditions have not been regarded as being within the sphere of neuromuscular rehabilitation; however, they should be. These conditions have an important motor component in their development (possibly) and persistence. Neuromuscular rehabilitation that encompasses cognitive and behavioural factors may have an important role to play in their management.[32–36]

From emotion and behaviour to pain

The non-traumatic pain condition is a curious entity. It was demonstrated that when a group of normal and healthy individuals is introduced to a manually repetitive task, within 6 months about a third develop a painful trapezius myalgia. This condition is further worsened if the individuals are experiencing psychological distress.[1–5,7–11,37–42] Repetitive low load work and psychological distress can each be a factor that leads to the development of this painful condition.[43] However, when combined, their effect seems to be magnified. The question is: how can pain and movement losses develop without an injury?

One of the most persistent findings is the individual's inability to relax their muscles during and after the performance of work-related tasks,[4,7,22,24,37,38,44–48] during time off work or leisure activities.[2,37,38,45]

During any given task there are periods when the muscles "switch off" or have very low level motor activity. These have been termed *rest gaps* or *relative rest periods* (Fig. 9.2). Generally, symptomatic individuals have overall reduced rest periods and there is a relationship between loss of rest gaps and an increase in pain levels and loss of range.[45,46,48–50]

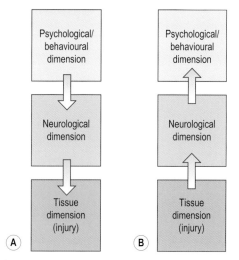

Fig. 9.1 • The aetiology and progression of **A**, non-traumatic pain conditions and **B**, musculoskeletal injury.

Individuals who are not in pain and who display such patterns of muscle activation are believed to be at an increased risk of developing trapezius myalgia.[2,37,38] Lundberg, who has done much research in this area, states, "it is possible that lack of relaxation is an even more important health problem than is the absolute level of contraction or the frequency of muscular activation".[2]

It seems that individuals "learn" a dysfunctional motor pattern which they habitually use during times of psychological distress or increased repetitive physical demands.[51] The individual may be unaware that they are tensing their muscles.[52–54] When these dysfunctional motor patterns become habitual they can be more resistant to change and tend to recur in the same muscle groups: the tension holding becomes autonomous (Ch. 2).[51,55] The person will have to be brought back to the cognitive

phase of motor learning in order to modify these patterns. The management would focus on relaxation ability using the principles of motor learning (see below and Ch. 3).

There seems to be a general trend to tense muscles in the upper part of the body and less caudally or in the limbs. Upper trapezius and frontalis were found to be the most common areas for muscle tension.[56,57] This may account for the high frequency of chronic pain conditions seen in the upper body such as trapezius myalgia, chronic pain around the scapula, upper thorax and neck pain.[2,11]

The inability to relax may also be present in musculoskeletal conditions where there is a history of injury. In chronic whiplash disorders it has been found that some of the muscle pain is associated with an inability to relax.[47] This tension may be related to the traumatic nature of the injury or in response to ongoing pain.

Changes in the muscle

The lack of rest periods may eventually lead to muscle-fibre damage, circulatory changes and pain.[1–3,56–59] Much of these changes takes place in the "slow twitch" (type I) muscle fibres, supplied by a low threshold motor unit.[60] During muscle contraction these units are the first to be activated and the last to switch off (Fig. 9.3).[61–63] It means that even during low-level physical activity, psychological stress or under high cognitive demands, these units would be continuously active.[64]

A frequent finding in biopsies taken directly from the tender points demonstrates focal muscle fibre damage, as well as grossly hypertrophied type I muscle fibres.[25,43,65,66,67,68] These are all indications that the muscle fibre is under excessive mechanical stress

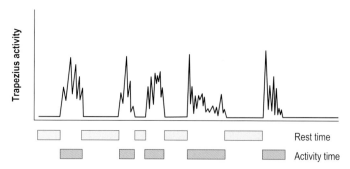

Fig. 9.2 • Rest and burst periods during trapezius muscle activity. Loss of rest period is often associated with trapezius myalgia.

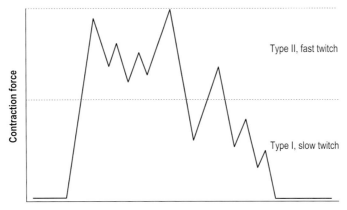

Fig. 9.3 • The Cinderella fibres. Type II slow twitch muscle fibres tend to be active throughout the contraction cycle. These fibres are more likely to show damage and hypertrophy in trapezius myalgia.

and undergoing cycles of injury and incomplete regeneration (Fig. 9.4).[22,24,25,69] The damage to cell membranes is associated with a release of pain-promoting substances locally and within the central nervous system (CNS).[70,71]

Another important finding is of reduced microcirculation to the damaged fibres as well as indications of energy crisis within the muscle cell.[65,67,71–75] This reduced flow impairs oxygen delivery and removal of metabolites in the working muscles and, consequently, will result in muscle pain.[65]

The areas of damage are associated with an increase in pressure-sensitive points in the muscle.[76,77] Repetitive activity or exercise tends to increase the pressure sensitivity and raises the level of pain.[70] The patient

often assumes that this pain is due to the muscle's being further damaged and inflamed. However, the non-traumatic pain conditions are not considered to be inflammatory disorders.[78] There are no inflammatory cells in the damaged muscle fibres or tender points. It only feels like that to the patient.

Message to the patient regarding non-traumatic pain conditions

- They are associated with only minor (but painful) changes in the muscles.
- There is low-level damage that is reversible.
- You can exercise as much as you want. It might be uncomfortable but you will not increase the damage.
- The pain is not due to inflammation. Anti-inflammatory medications are unlikely to help.

Normal fibres

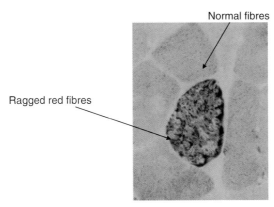

Ragged red fibres

Fig. 9.4 • Local muscle fibre damage in trapezius myalgia. (From Larssona B, Bjorka J, Henriksson KG, Gerdleb B, Lindmand R 2000 The prevalence of cytochrome c oxidase negative and superpositive fibres and ragged-red fibres in the trapezius muscle of female cleaners with and without myalgia and of female healthy controls. Pain 84:379–387, with permission.)

A secondary hypersensitivity pain condition?

Part of the experience of pain in the non-traumatic condition may be associated with a secondary hypersensitivity process. Such hypersensitivity often develops as a consequence of an ongoing experience of pain.[31,79,80]

In essence, the longer a certain nociceptive pathway is active, the more its threshold is reduced and the more it becomes sensitized (like a well-trodden path, Fig. 9.5). It is an adaptive process; a "pain learning or imprinting" phenomenon that occurs throughout

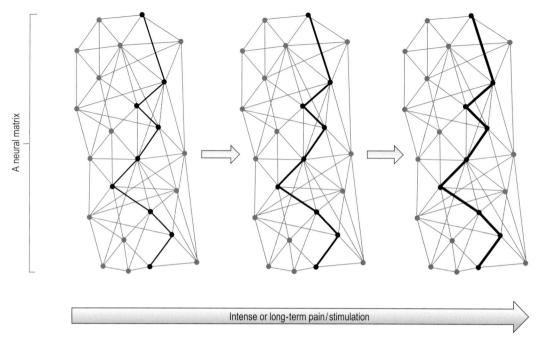

A neural matrix

Intense or long-term pain/stimulation

Fig. 9.5 • Pain imprinting. Prolonged or intense pain experiences may lead to central sensitization.

the CNS (often termed *central sensitization*).[81–89] Consequently, as time passes, even minor events in the person's life may trigger disproportionately greater pain experiences (Fig. 9.6).[88,90]

Once the sensitization has taken place it is does not seem to be dependent any longer on nociception from the damaged tissue; it is now an autonomous pain condition.[91] The pain condition now "resides" within the CNS and is more open to influence by other central processes, such as the moods, emotions and cognitions of the individual.

Managing non-traumatic pain conditions

It was once believed that patients suffering from non-traumatic pain conditions were suffering from localized muscle pathology. The therapeutic focus was in the periphery, targeting the painful muscle. The treatment often consisted of muscle stretching, massage, muscle energy technique, trying to switch off trigger points, and various forms of exercise. In my clinical experience many of these treatments have some effect, but with diminishing returns. The effects would only last for a short time; the patients remained in a chronic state of pain.[92–94]

It was demonstrated that even the injection of botulinum toxin into the painful muscles (a toxin that causes muscle paralysis) has only a temporary effect lasting about 3 months.[19] This study carries an important clinical message. The therapeutic attention should move away from treating the periphery – the muscle or the symptoms of the conditions. But where should the focus be?

In the last decade the role of psychological–behavioural processes in these conditions has became more evident (Fig. 9.7). These studies indicate that we should be focusing on these processes ("the person") and away from treating the periphery (the muscle). A more successful clinical outcome can be achieved by workplace changes, providing the patient with a better understanding of their condition, promoting self-care and engaging the patient's coping strategies.[95–97] Within this management, the patient can be trained to relax the tense and painful areas (see below).

Working with cognitions: changing the narrative

When individuals are in pain or have an injury, their beliefs about and attitudes towards their conditions are constructed into an internal narrative. They may

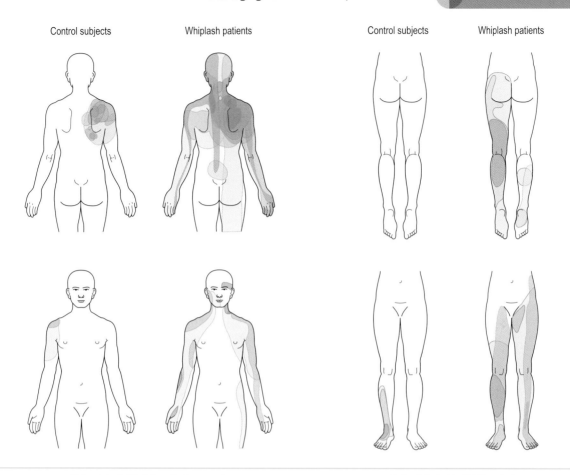

Control subjects   Whiplash patients   Control subjects   Whiplash patients

Saline injected to infraspinatus muscle   **Saline injected to tibialis anterior**

Fig. 9.6 • Central sensitization in chronic whiplash syndrome. Injection of an irritant into the muscle results in wide-spread sensitivity. (From Koelbaek Johansen M 1999 Generalised muscular hyperalgesia in chronic whiplash syndrome. Pain 83(2):229–234, with permission).

contain messages that the pain is due to a serious pathological process affecting the muscles and/or joints in the neck; that the condition is permanent and non-reversible and will result in some neck movement disability. Many patients will withdraw from physical activities believing that they are inflicting further damage on their painful tissues. These attitudes and beliefs hold them back from taking positive actions that could help them to improve.

Providing the patients with an alternative narrative can help to reassure and empower them. The alternative narrative can include information about possible underlying processes associated with these conditions.[95–97] They can be informed that it is not a pathological condition in the muscle, that pain is not necessarily an indication of damage and that the

damage is microscopically small. Since muscle repairs and regenerates very quickly, once the causes are removed the muscle is expected to recover fully. It will not leave permanent damage, and physical activity, although painful, does not increase the damage.

Sometimes raising the patient's awareness and bringing their attention to the sensations in their body in relation to what they feel can be helpful. Some patients believe that somehow their muscles "tense on them". They might not be aware that they tense their own muscles and that they may be able to control the level of tension. The management aims to bring the patient's awareness to the situations where tension rises, as well as exploring with the patient some coping strategies that would help them to relax.

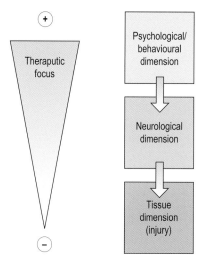

Fig. 9.7 • In the non-traumatic pain condition the therapeutic focus should be towards the psychological–behavioural dimension of the individual. Treatment of the symptomatic muscle, in the tissue dimension, is unlikely to provide long-term solutions. It is attempting to resolve the condition from the periphery by focusing on the condition's symptoms rather than its causes.

Working with behaviours

Several work-related factors are associated with trapezius myalgia and chronic neck pain. These include work postures that involve long periods of neck and arm use in awkward postures, particularly when the arm is used above shoulder level. Further risk factors are repetitive bending and twisting of the upper spine/neck and sedentary work for more than 5 hours a day.[39,98–100]

We can see from the above that preventive intervention has to be in both the task and organizational spheres of behaviour (Ch. 8). Task-behaviour is the way people use their body in relation to objects. The working posture should be assessed and advice given where risk factors are identified (if necessary patients can get themselves photographed at work using their mobile phones and bring the photo(s) to the session). Organizational behaviour was identified as the way people organize their tasks into complex routines. Minor modifications, such as the introduction of rest periods, reducing the duration of sitting and/or alternating it with other non-sedentary tasks may be helpful. Even adding physical exercise during work has been shown to have a positive effect on neck and shoulder complaints.[101]

During periods of stress and/or increased workload individuals may be drawn away from coping strategies that could help them to unwind and self-care. For example, sedentary workers with low levels of leisure-time activity had a higher prevalence of neck disorders.[102] It is useful to identify these coping strategies and encourage the patient to reintroduce them into their routines. Unwinding can be a form of leisure activity such as – reading, sports, exercise, playing a musical instrument, meditation or yoga; any activity that brings the person "back to themselves". Avoid imposing your own coping strategies on the patient, find out what works for them.

Mind over motor: use of relaxation ability

In the last few years the trend has been to introduce exercise to individuals suffering from chronic neck pain and trapezius myalgia, despite the finding that there are associations with an inability to relax and overuse syndrome. Very little research has been carried out to assess the therapeutic value of relaxation.[103,104,105]

Relaxation is a motor learning process and, therefore, practice should incorporate the five code elements for neuromuscular adaptation: cognition, being active, feedback, repetition and the similarity principle (Ch. 5).

In my experience the approach that had a major positive therapeutic effect was the introduction of "focused motor relaxation" and integrating it with the adaptation code. In this approach the patient is trained to direct relaxation to the specific painful areas. This learning can be achieved by different means: focused relaxation, contract–relax or gentle elongation to encourage letting go.

Focused motor relaxation could commence on the treatment table with the therapist palpating the patient's neck and shoulder, focusing on areas where the patients feels pain and stiffness. Using the hands the therapist provides the patient with manual or verbal feedback, guiding the patient through a process of *focused motor relaxation* (cognitive element). Where tender and stiff areas in the head/neck/shoulder are found, the patient is prompted to "soften" them (active element). An immediate and continuous feedback about the state of the muscle is verbally conveyed to the patient (feedback element). Once the patient is able to relax a particular area, the therapist can move on to other symptomatic areas, carrying out this search-and-relax procedure. The search-and-relax procedure is repeated several times during the same and subsequent treatments (repetition element).

The contract–relax method can be added to bring awareness to muscles that patients find difficult to relax. The patient is instructed to "tense" the affected area, followed by a *slow* relaxation. During the slow relaxation the patient is made aware of the sensation of relaxation in the muscle. Gentle passive elongation can also be used to give a sense of length in the shortened, tense muscle. During this manoeuvre the patient can experience the "letting go": how the muscle is relaxing and elongating. (It is not a stretching technique for the muscle.)

Missing in this approach is the similarity principle. Relaxation training on the treatment table is dissimilar to relaxation during upright posture and various upper-body tasks. It is also out of context to the place and situation in which the patient experiences the tension (e.g. work).[30] Hence, the relaxation training should be practised in the postures that are associated with the pain and tension. For example, computer users are invited to sit in the typing position (I have a keyboard in the clinic for that purpose). While the patient is writing or typing, the therapist applies the search-and-relax procedure on the neck and shoulders. Verbal and manual feedback is used to guide the relaxation process. The shoulders and neck are guided into positions that suggest the individual is relaxing (e.g. dropping the shoulders).

The patients are encouraged to transfer the relaxation experience to their daily activities: a *functional relaxation*. The aim is to achieve movement patterns in which there is minimal tension and optimal energy efficiency. This functional relaxation combined with biofeedback was demonstrated to increase the trapezius relative rest time during computer work.[106] This approach is akin to the relaxation-in-movement used in the Alexander method. A recent study has shown that six lessons in Alexander technique combined with exercise (mostly walking) achieved long-term improvements for back pain sufferers.[107]

Managing the painful jaw

A similar focused motor relaxation approach can be used to manage patients suffering from muscular jaw pain (bruxism). This condition is marked by an increased clenching of the jaw and grinding of the teeth, mainly during the night, resulting in muscle pain and even in tooth and temporomandibular joint damage.[20,21] Painful jaw condition is also associated with psychological stress and anxiety states and shares many of the processes seen in trapezius myalgia, including the loss of relaxation ability.[12–17,24]

The same neuromuscular approach described above is used for managing patients suffering from jaw pain: focused motor relaxation using the search–relax method while palpating the different face/jaw muscles. The patient is guided to "make their jaw heavy" and "let the teeth separate". This is combined with gentle elongation, dropping of the lower jaw. For the similarity principle the patient is encouraged to transfer the sense of relaxation to daily situations and to three key points during the night: just as they fall asleep, during the night and immediately upon waking-up (there is some evidence of nocturnal spontaneous muscle activity in patients with lower back pain and patients with chronic trapezius myalgia).[54,108]

There are several focused relaxation exercises that can be given to the patient. They should remind themselves during the day to make the "jaw heavy" and to try to keep their upper and lower teeth slightly separated to prevent clenching. Another is to pronounce the sound "baaa" (not to be practised in the presence of sheep). This may seem very silly, but it encourages relaxation of the "clenchers" of the jaw. Once the jaw is relaxed the patient should be able to hold it and move it freely from side to side. This can be used by the patient to assess their ability to relax the jaw.

A note on relaxation ability

Patients with chronic tension headaches and lower back pain are less able to discriminate between the different levels of muscle tension at the painful area.[109] They generally overestimate low and underestimate high levels of muscle tension. For this group relaxation training for tension headache was found to be less effective.[110]

Perhaps in this group of patients we should be looking at improving the cognitive abilities of introspection and discrimination?

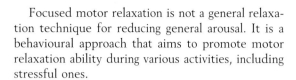

Focused motor relaxation is not a general relaxation technique for reducing general arousal. It is a behavioural approach that aims to promote motor relaxation ability during various activities, including stressful ones.

Non-traumatic pain: the injury response and exercise

In the non-traumatic conditions the nervous system may initiate an injury response related to the individual's experience of pain. This response is often disproportionate to the underlying damage, which is often minimal. As such, the parametric abilities and synergistic control are likely to be affected. Indeed, losses in some of these abilities have been demonstrated in chronic neck conditions.[44,45] However, it should be noted that these changes are more likely to be the outcome of the condition than the cause. There is no association between low muscle strength, low muscle endurance, and reduced spinal mobility for developing neck pain (also lower back pain).[111]

Exercise for non-traumatic pain conditions

The injury response to the experience of pain has led several groups to develop neck and shoulder exercises to overcome these control changes.

Several studies have demonstrated some benefit from various forms of exercise in the reduction of the symptoms of trapezius myalgia.[103,112–116] These include strength and/or endurance training,[117] non-specific general exercise and specific neck exercises.[35,118] Interestingly, also useful were Qigong and coordination exercises, which promote relaxation and movement efficiency.[36,114,115,119] However, exercise is only of limited benefit when compared to other interventions (massage, ergonomic advice),[93,94] and their effects tend to diminish over time.[115] In order to sustain some effect, the individual would have to maintain a punishing, ongoing exercise regime.

Treating the consequences, i.e. the symptoms, may provide temporary relief, but does not solve the underlying problem – exercise by itself is not motor rehabilitation. The person will "learn" the specific exercise control, but it will not transfer to control for daily functional patterns.[120] This is important, as it became fashionable to apply the core stability type training to the neck. This includes using "the hammer" of force and endurance to beat the system into shape. It is often accompanied by exercise that aims to modify the onset timing of the deep and superficial neck muscle using the erroneous concept of focusing on particular muscles and extra-functional movement patterns. Such approaches do not transfer to control of normal functional neck movement.[120]

It is curious why exercise should have a positive effect for individuals who are suffering from an overuse condition and an inability to relax. Furthermore, how it is that such different exercise approaches have a positive effect? Generally, when everything seems to work, something else is happening. Probably the main reason for improvement with exercise is to do with psychological factors that include empowerment of the patient, reducing fear of use and providing a proactive coping strategy to pain. This phenomenon is seen in patients with chronic back pain, where all forms of exercise seem to be equally effective in improving this condition.[121]

It is also possible that exercise has a modifying effect on pain mechanisms associated with central sensitization rather than eliminating the causes. Another possibility is that, exercise may bring about adaptive changes that reverse some of the damage seen in the affected muscle fibres[73,122–124] as well as helping to re-establish normal perfusion to the damaged fibres.[125–128] However, all the physiological effects of exercise are likely to be temporary if the patient stops exercising and the underlying causes are not dealt with.

A neuromuscular rehabilitation approach to neck exercise

Any exercise can be used for reassurance, including the ones described above. However, these exercises are dissimilar to normal neck movement. Most functional head movements are non-contact, whereas resistance exercises are all in contact (Ch. 2). Also the head follows our senses or leads in certain activities such as walking and turning. Hence, it might be more beneficial to challenge neck control in contact-free and goal-orientated movement.

This control can be challenged, for example, by instructing the patient to draw imaginary numbers in space leading with the tip of their nose (Fig. 9.8,a,b&c). Sets of numbers from 0 to 10 can be used in different head positions (Fig. 9.8a). During the exercise the patient is instructed to relax their neck and shoulder muscles and to attempt to perform the movement as smoothly as possible. This is to account for the finding that patients with chronic neck pain tend to have more "jerky" neck movements (due to reduced coordination and synergistic abilities).[129]

Another exercise is to repetitively nod the head in a "Yes-Yes" (Fig. 9.8b), "No-No" (Fig. 9.8c) patterns throughout the range of rotation (see Video, part 3).

Clinical notes on passive and active approaches

So what should we prescribe to our patients, exercise or relaxation or both? A pragmatic approach is needed here. Basically, try one approach and if it does not produce the expected results, move on to another.

Generally, start with a relaxation approach and the number-counting exercise. This approach requires the least commitment of time and effort from the patient, and it can be easily applied at work or in stressful situations. This approach could be useful if the patient is suffering from high levels of pain. The active approach/exercise may be left out if the patient improves and shows signs that the relaxation approach is sufficient for maintaining the improvement (I would usually expect improvement within 3–6 weeks).

If the patient is not showing signs of improvement then use an exercise approach. This can be introduced in a gradual manner, using some of the techniques described above.

If the patient has a history of exercising, they should be encouraged to return to their sporting activities. They are also more likely to take on any exercise given by the therapist. If the patient has no such history they are unlikely to adhere to exercise. In this case the therapist may return to the relaxation option. This, of course, does not exclude the concurrent use of relaxation and exercise approaches.

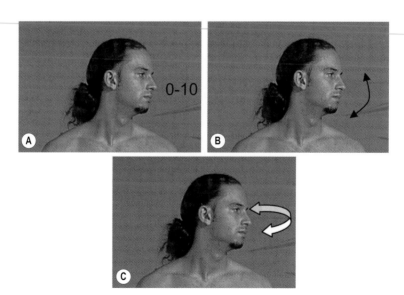

Fig. 9.8 • Challenging movement control of the neck. In all the procedures the patient is instructed to relax their shoulder and neck, and to perform the movement as smoothly as possible. **A**, drawing imaginary numbers from 0 to 10 at the end range of rotation. **B**, Small amplitude "Yes-Yes" movement and **C**, Patient is instructed to perform repetitive, small amplitude "No-No" movement patterns at the end range.

Summary points

- Individuals may acquire painful musculoskeletal conditions without injury.
- Often these conditions develop in low-load, repetitive physical activities (e.g. using a computer).
- They may also develop in response to psychological distress.
- These conditions often manifest as pain and tender points around the head (tension headache), suboccipital area, neck and neck-scapular muscles (trapezius myalgia) and jaw (bruxism).
- Probably some forms of non-specific lower back pain are also associated with this group of conditions.
- All these conditions share similar processes: inability of the individual to relax, transmission of tension via the neuromuscular system to specific muscles, hypertrophy and damage of specific muscle fibres and disturbance to microcirculation, and release of pain-related substances locally.
- A secondary, central pain sensitization may play an important role in the pain experience.

- Intervention should be all-inclusive – a combination of cognitive, psychosocial, behavioural and neuromuscular approaches.
- The aim in the cognitive dimension is to reassure and empower the patient to self-care.
- In the behavioural dimension the individual should be assessed and guided in their task and organizational behaviour.
- Focused motor relaxation should be used to train the individual in how to relax their painful muscles/areas.
- Focused motor relaxation is a motor learning experience. It is not about reducing arousal.
- Transferring the relaxation to functional daily activities is important. Promote relaxation-in-movement.
- The patient's own coping strategies are very important for reducing stress and chronic states of arousal.
- Exercise can provide temporary relief from pain. However, it has only limited and short-lasting effect.
- Pain cannot be beaten into submission! Avoid punishing exercise regimes and avoid painful manual techniques.
- Neuromuscular rehabilitation is also about motor relaxation.

References

[1] Lundberg U, Dohns IE, Melin B, et al. Psychophysiological stress responses, muscle tension, and neck and shoulder pain among supermarket cashiers. J Occup Health Psychol 1999;4(3): 245–255.

[2] Lundberg U. Stress responses in low-status jobs and their relationship to health risks: musculoskeletal disorders. Ann NY Acad Sci 1999;896:162–172.

[3] Lundberg U. Psychological stress and musculoskeletal disorders: psychobiological mechanisms. Lack of rest and recovery greater problem than workload. Lakartidningen 2003;100(21): 1892–1895.

[4] Sandsjo L, Melin B, Rissen D, et al. Trapezius muscle activity, neck and shoulder pain, and subjective experiences during monotonous work in women. Eur J Appl Physiol 2000;83(2–3): 235–238.

[5] Nordander C, Hansson GA, Rylander L, et al. Muscular rest and gap frequency as EMG measures of physical exposure: the impact of work tasks and individual related factors. Ergonomics 2000;43(11): 1904–1919.

[6] Holte KA, Westgaard RH. Further studies of shoulder and neck pain and exposures in customer service work with low biomechanical demands. Ergonomics 2002;45(13): 887–909.

[7] Holte KA, Westgaard RH. Daytime trapezius muscle activity and shoulder-neck pain of service workers with work stress and low biomechanical exposure. Am J Indust Med 2002;41(5):393–405.

[8] Larsson B, Bjork J, Elert J, et al. Mechanical performance and electromyography during repeated maximal isokinetic shoulder forward flexions in female cleaners with and without myalgia of the trapezius muscle and in healthy controls. Eur J Appl Physiol 2000;83(4–5): 257–267.

[9] Hoogendoorn WE, Bongers PM, de Vet HC, et al. High physical work load and low job satisfaction increase the risk of sickness absence due to low back pain: results of a prospective cohort study. Occup Environ Health Med 2003;59(5): 323–328.

[10] Ariens GA, Bongers PM, Hoogendoorn WE, et al. High quantitative job demands and low coworker support as risk factors for neck pain: results of a

prospective cohort study. Spine 2001;26(17):1896–1901.

[11] Ariens GA, Bongers PM, Hoogendoorn WE, et al. High physical and psychosocial load at work and sickness absence due to neck pain. Scand J Work Environ Health 2002;28(4):222–231.

[12] Lobbezoo F, Naeije M. Bruxism is mainly regulated centrally, not peripherally. J Oral Rehabil 2001;28(12):1085–1091.

[13] Mikami DB. A review of psychogenic aspects and treatment of bruxism. J Prosthet Dent 1977;37(4):411–419.

[14] Flor H, Birbaumer N, Schulte W, et al. Stress-related electromyographic responses in patients with chronic temporomandibular pain. Pain 1991;46(2):145–152.

[15] Thompson BA, Blount BW, Krumholz TS. Treatment approaches to bruxism. Am Fam Physician 1994;49(7):1617–1622.

[16] Restrepo CC, Alvarez E, Jaramillo C, et al. Effects of psychological techniques on bruxism in children with primary teeth. J Oral Rehabil 2001; 28(4):354–360.

[17] Dahlstrom L, Carlsson SG, Gale EN, et al. Stress-induced muscular activity in mandibular dysfunction: effects of biofeedback training. J Behav Med 1985;8(2):191–200.

[18] Holmgren K, Sheikholeslam A, Riise C, et al. The effects of an occlusal splint on the electromyographic activities of the temporal and masseter muscles during maximal clenching in patients with a habit of nocturnal bruxism and signs and symptoms of craniomandibular disorders. J Oral Rehabil 1990;17(5): 447–459.

[19] To EW, Ahuja AT, Ho WS, et al. A prospective study of the effect of botulinum toxin A on masseteric muscle hypertrophy with ultrasonographic and electromyographic measurement. BJPS 2001;54(3):197–200.

[20] Wieselmann G, Permann R, Korner E, et al. Nocturnal sleep studies of bruxism. EEG-EMG EEG EMG Z Elektroenzephalogr

Elektromyogr Verwandte Geb 1986;17(1):32–36.

[21] Rugh JD, Harlan J. Nocturnal bruxism and temporomandibular disorders. Adv Neurol 1988;49:329–341.

[22] Satoh K, Yamaguchi T, Komatsu K, et al. Analyses of muscular activity, energy metabolism, and muscle fiber type composition in a patient with bilateral masseteric hypertrophy. Cranio 2001; 19(4):294–301.

[23] Hamada T, Kotani H, Kawazoe Y, et al. Effect of occlusal splints on the EMG activity of masseter and temporal muscles in bruxism with clinical symptoms. J Oral Rehabil 1982;9(2):119–123.

[24] McGlynn FD, Bichajian C, Tira DE, et al. The effect of experimental stress and experimental occlusal interference on masseteric EMG activity. J Cranio Dis 1989;3(2): 87–92.

[25] Newton JP, Cowpe JG, McClure IJ, et al. Masseteric hypertrophy? preliminary report. J Oral Maxillo Surg 1999;37(5): 405–408.

[26] Jensen R. Pathophysiology of headache. Pathophysiol 1998; 5(1):196.

[27] Altura BM, Altura BT. Tension headaches and muscle tension: is there a role for magnesium? Med Hypoth 2001;57(6):705–713.

[28] Rokicki LA, Holroyd KA, France CR, et al. Change mechanisms associated with combined relaxation/EMG biofeedback training for chronic tension headache. Appl Psychophysiol Biofeedback 1997;22(1):21–41.

[29] Arena JG, Bruno GM, Hannah SL, et al. A comparison of frontal electromyographic biofeedback training, trapezius electromyographic biofeedback training, and progressive muscle relaxation therapy in the treatment of tension headache. Headache 1995;35(7):411–419.

[30] Reeves JL. EMG-biofeedback reduction of tension headache: a cognitive skills-training approach. Biofeedback Self Regul 1976; 1(2):217–225.

[31] Fernández-de-Las-Peñas C, Ge HY, Arendt-Nielsen L, et al. Referred pain from trapezius muscle trigger points shares similar characteristics with chronic tension type headache. Eur J Pain 2007;11(4):475–482 Epub 2006 Aug 21.

[32] Ingeborg BC, Bos Korthals-de, Hoving JL, et al. Cost effectiveness of physiotherapy, manual therapy, and general practitioner care for neck pain: economic evaluation alongside a randomised controlled trial. BMJ 2003;326:911.

[33] De Laat A, Stappaerts K, Papy S. Counseling and physical therapy as treatment for myofascial pain of the masticatory system. J Orofac Pain 2003;17(1):42–49.

[34] Goffaux-Dogniez C, Vanfraechem-Raway R, Verbanck P. Appraisal of treatment of the trigger points associated with relaxation to treat chronic headache in the adult. Relationship with anxiety and stress adaptation strategies. L'Encephale 2003;29(5):377–390.

[35] Blangsted AK, Søgaard K, Hansen EA, et al. One-year randomized controlled trial with different physical-activity programs to reduce musculoskeletal symptoms in the neck and shoulders among office workers. Scand J Work Environ Health 2008;34(1):55–65.

[36] Lansinger B, Larsson E, Persson LC, et al. Qigong and exercise therapy in patients with long-term neck pain: a prospective randomized trial. Spine 2007;32(22):2415–2422.

[37] Veiersted KB, Westgaard RH, Andersen P. Pattern of muscle activity during stereotyped work and its relation to muscle pain. Int Arch Occup Environ Health 1990;62(1):31–41.

[38] Veiersted KB, Westgaard RH, Andersen P. Electromyographic evaluation of muscular work pattern as a predictor of trapezius myalgia. Scand. J. Work Environ. Health 1993;19(4):284–290.

[39] Walker-Bone K, Palmer KT, Reading I, et al. Soft-tissue rheumatic disorders of the neck and upper limb: prevalence and

risk factors. Semin Arthritis Rheum 2003;33(3):185–203.

[40] Houtman IL, Bongers PM, Smulders PG, et al. Psychosocial stressors at work and musculoskeletal problems. Scand J Work, Environ Health 1994; 20(2):139–145.

[41] Roe C, Bjorklund RA, Knardahl S, et al. Cognitive performance and muscle activation in workers with chronic shoulder myalgia. Ergonomics 2001;44(1):1–16.

[42] Hasenbring M, Hallner D, Klasen B. Psychological mechanisms in the transition from acute to chronic pain: over- or underrated? Schmerz 2001;15(6):442–447.

[43] Andersen LL, Suetta C, Andersen JL, et al. Increased proportion of megafibers in chronically painful muscles. Pain Aug 2008;11: [Epub ahead of print].

[44] Johnston V, Jull G, Souvlis T, et al. Neck movement and muscle activity characteristics in female office workers with neck pain. Spine 2008;33(5):555–563.

[45] Johnston V, Jull G, Darnell R, et al. Alterations in cervical muscle activity in functional and stressful tasks in female office workers with neck pain. Eur J Appl Physiol 2008;103(3): 253–264 Epub 2008 Feb 22.

[46] Frankenhaeuser M, Lundberg U, Fredrikson M, et al. Stress on and off the job as related to sex and occupational status in white-collar workers. J Organiz Behavior 1989;10:321–346.

[47] Elert J, Kendall SA, Larsson B, et al. Chronic pain and difficulty in relaxing postural muscles in patients with fibromyalgia and chronic whiplash associated disorders. J Rheumatol 2001; 28(6):1361–1368.

[48] Thorn S, Søgaard K, Kallenberg LA, et al. Trapezius muscle rest time during standardised computer work – a comparison of female computer users with and without self-reported neck/shoulder complaints. J Electromyogr Kinesiol 2007;17(4):420–427.

[49] Mork PJ, Westgaard RH. Low-amplitude trapezius activity in work and leisure and the relation to shoulder and neck pain. J Appl Physiol 2006; 100(4):1142–1149.

[50] Goudy N, McLean L. Using myoelectric signal parameters to distinguish between computer workers with and without trapezius myalgia. Eur J Appl Physiol 2006;97(2):196–209.

[51] Schneider C, Palomba D, Flor H. Pavlovian conditioning of muscular responses in chronic pain patients: central and peripheral correlates. Pain 2004;112(3):239–247.

[52] Jonsson B. Measurement and evaluation of local muscular strain in the shoulder during constrained work. J Hum Ergol 1982;11:73–88.

[53] Westgaard R. Measurement and evaluation of postural load in occupational work situations. Eur J Appl Physiol 1988;57(3): 291–304.

[54] Westgaard RH, Bonato P, Holte KA. Low-frequency oscillations (<0.3 Hz) in the electromyographic (EMG) activity of the human trapezius muscle during sleep. J Neurophysiol 2002;88(3): 1177–1184.

[55] Flor H, Birbaumer N, Schugens MM, Lutzenberger W. Symptom-specific psychophysiological responses in chronic pain patients. Psychophysiol 1992;29(4): 452–460.

[56] Waersted M, Westgaard RH. Attention-related muscle activity in different body regions during VDU work with minimal physical activity. Ergonomics 1996;39(4): 661–676.

[57] Waersted M. Human muscle activity related to non-biomechanical factors in the workplace. Eur J Appl Physiol 2000;83(2–3):151–158.

[58] Holte KA, Vasseljen O, Westgaard RH. Exploring perceived tension as a response to psychosocial work stress. Scand J Work, Environ Health 2003; 29(2):124–133.

[59] Kitahara T, Schnoz M, Laubli T, et al. Motor-unit activity in the trapezius muscle during rest, while inputting data, and during fast finger tapping. Eur J Appl Physiol 2000;83(2–3):181–189.

[60] Henneman E. Skeletal muscle: the servant of the nervous system. In: Mountcastle VB, editor. Medical physiology. 14th ed. St Louis: Mosby; 1980. p. 674–680.

[61] Conwit RA, Stashuk D, Tracy B, et al. The relationship of motor unit size, firing rate and force. Clin Neurophysiol 1999;110 (7):1270–1275.

[62] Hagg G. Static work loads and occupational myalgia – a new explanation model. In: Anderson PA, Hobart DJ, Danhoff JV, editors. Electromyographical kinesiology. London: Elsevier Science; 1991. p. 141–144.

[63] Kadefors R, Forsman M, Zoega B, et al. Recruitment of low threshold motor-units in the trapezius muscle in different static arm positions. Ergonomics 1999;42(2):359–375.

[64] Waersted M, Eken T, Westgaard RH. Activity of single motor units in attention-demanding tasks: firing pattern in the human trapezius muscle. Eur J Appl Physiol Occup Physiol 1996;72(4):323–329.

[65] Kadi F, Waling K, Ahlgren C, et al. Pathological mechanisms implicated in localized female trapezius myalgia. Pain 1998; 78(3):191–196.

[66] Larsson B, Bjork J, Henriksson KG, et al. The prevalences of cytochrome c oxidase negative and superpositive fibres and ragged-red fibres in the trapezius muscle of female cleaners with and without myalgia and of female healthy controls. Pain 2000;84(2–3):379–387.

[67] Larsson SE, Bengtsson A, Bodegard L, et al. Muscle changes in work-related chronic myalgia. Acta Orthop Scand 1988; 59(5):552–556.

[68] Larsson B, Bjork J, Elert J, Lindman R, Gerdle B. Fibre type proportion and fibre size in trapezius muscle biopsies from cleaners with and without myalgia and its correlation with ragged red fibres, cytochrome-c-oxidase-negative fibres, biomechanical output, perception of fatigue, and

surface electromyography during repetitive forward flexions. Eur J Appl Physiol 2001;84(6): 492–502.

[69] Kadi F, Hagg G, Hakansson R, et al. Structural changes in male trapezius muscle with work-related myalgia. Acta Neuropathol (Berl) 1998;95(4):352–360.

[70] Rosendale L, Larsson B, Kristiansen J, et al. Increase in muscle nociceptive substances and anaerobic metabolism in patients with trapezius myalgia: microdialysis in rest and during exercise. Pain 2004;112:324–334.

[71] Larsson R, Oberg PA, Larsson SE. Changes of trapezius muscle blood flow and electromyography in chronic neck pain due to trapezius myalgia. Pain 1999; 79(1):45–50.

[72] Lindman R, Hagberg M, Angqvist KA, et al. Changes in muscle morphology in chronic trapezius myalgia. Scand J Work Environ Health 1991;17(5): 347–355.

[73] Larsson SE, Bodegard L, Henriksson KG, et al. Chronic trapezius myalgia. Morphology and blood flow studied in 17 patients. Acta Orthop Scand 1990;61(5):394–398.

[74] Larsson R, Cai H, Zhang Q, et al. Visualization of chronic neck-shoulder pain: impaired microcirculation in the upper trapezius muscle in chronic cervico-brachial pain. Occup Med (Oxford, England) 1998;48(3): 189–194.

[75] Ashina M, Stallknecht B, Bendtsen L, et al. In vivo evidence of altered skeletal muscle blood flow in chronic tension-type headache. Brain 2002;125 (Part 2):320–326.

[76] Leffler AS, Hansson P, Kosek E. Somatosensory perception in patients suffering from long-term trapezius myalgia at the site overlying the most painful part of the muscle and in an area of pain referral. Eur J Pain 2003;7(3): 267–276.

[77] Hagg GM, Astrom A. Load pattern and pressure pain threshold in the upper trapezius muscle and psychosocial factors in medical secretaries with and without shoulder/neck disorders. Int Arch Occup Environ Health 1997;69(6):423–432.

[78] Ashina M, Stallknecht B, Bendtsen L, Pedersen JF, Schifter S, Galbo H, et al. Tender points are not sites of ongoing inflammation – in vivo evidence in patients with chronic tension-type headache. Cephalalgia 2003;23(2):109–116.

[79] Buchgreitz L, Lyngberg AC, Bendtsen L, et al. Frequency of headache is related to sensitization: a population study. Pain 2006;123(1–2):19–27.

[80] Yokoyama T, Lisi TL, Moore SA, et al. Muscle fatigue increases the probability of developing hyperalgesia in mice. J Pain 2007;8(9):692–699.

[81] Flor H, Braun C, Elbert T, et al. Extensive reorganization of primary somatosensory cortex in chronic back pain patients. Neurosci Lett 1997;224(1):5–8.

[82] Obata K, Noguchi K. MAPK activation in nociceptive neurons and pain hypersensitivity. Life Sci 2004;74(21):2643–2653.

[83] Zimmermann M. Neuronal mechanisms of chronic pain. Orthopade 2004;33(5): 515–524.

[84] Cook AJ, Woolf CJ, Wall PD, et al. Dynamic receptive field plasticity in rat spinal dorsal horn following C-primary afferent input. Nature 1987;325:151–153.

[85] Hylden JLK, Nahin RL, Traub RJ, et al. Expansion of receptive fields of spinal lamina I projection neurons in rat with unilateral adjuvant-induced inflammation: the contribution of dorsal horn mechanisms. Pain 1989;37:229–243.

[86] Dunbar R, Ruda MA. Activity-dependent neuronal plasticity following tissue injury and inflammation. Trends Neurosci 1992;15(3):96–103.

[87] Woolf CJ. The dorsal horn: state-dependent sensory processing and the generation of pain. In: Wall PD, Melzack R, editors. Textbook of pain. 3rd ed. London: Churchill Livingstone; 1994. p. 101–112.

[88] Woolf CJ, Salter MW. Neural plasticity: increasing the gain in pain. Science 2000;288:1765–1769.

[89] Millan MJ. Descending control of pain. Prog Neurobiol 2002; 66(6):355–474.

[90] Hoheisel U, Mense S, Simon DG. Appearance of new receptive fields in rat dorsal horn neurons following noxious stimulation of skeletal muscle. Neurosci 1993;153:9–12.

[91] Curatolo M, Petersen-Felix S, Arendt-Nielsen L, et al. Central hypersensitivity in chronic pain after whiplash injury. Clin J Pain 2001;17(4):306–315.

[92] Brewer S, Eerd DV, Amick IB, et al. Workplace interventions to prevent musculoskeletal and visual symptoms and disorders among computer users: a systematic review. J Occup Rehabil 2006;16(3):317–350.

[93] Verhagen AP, Karels C, Bierma-Zeinstra SMA, et al. 2006; Ergonomic and physiotherapeutic interventions for treating work-related complaints of the arm, neck or shoulder in adults. Cochrane Reviews (3) CD003471. doi:10.1002/ 14651858.CD003471.pub3.

[94] Verhagen AP, Karels C, Bierma-Zeinstra SM, Feleus A, Dahaghin S, Burdorf A, et al. Exercise proves effective in a systematic review of work related complaints of the arm, neck, or shoulder. J Clin Epidemiol 2007;60(2):110–117.

[95] Nederhand MJ, Ijzerman MJ, Hermens HJ, et al. Predictive value of fear avoidance in developing chronic neck pain disability: consequences for clinical decision making. Arch Phys Med Rehabil 2004;85(3): 496–501.

[96] Linton SJ, Andersson T. Can chronic disability be prevented? A randomized trial of a cognitive-behavior intervention and two forms of information for patients with spinal pain. Spine 2000; 25(21):2825–2831.

[97] Linton SJ, Ryberg M. A cognitive-behavioral group intervention as prevention for persistent neck and back pain in a non-patient population: a randomized controlled trial. Pain 2001; 90(1–2):83–90.

[98] Ariens GA, van Mechelen W, Bongers PM, et al. Physical risk factors for neck pain. Scand J Work Environ Health 2000; 26(1):7–19.

[99] van der Windt DA, Thomas E, Pope DP, et al. Occupational risk factors for shoulder pain: a systematic review. Occup Environ Med 2000;57(7): 433–442.

[100] Malchaire J, Cock N, Vergracht S. Review of the factors associated with musculoskeletal problems in epidemiological studies. Int Arch Occup Environ Health 2001;74(2):79–90.

[101] Proper KI, Koning M, Van der Beek AJ, et al. The effectiveness of worksite physical activity programs on physical activity, physical fitness, and health. Clin J Sport Med 2003;13(2): 106–117.

[102] Hildebrandt VH, Bongers PM, Dul J, et al. The relationship between leisure time, physical activities and musculoskeletal symptoms and disability in worker populations. Int Arch Occup Environ Health 2000; 73(8):507–518.

[103] Viljanen M, Malmivaara A, Uitti J, et al. Effectiveness of dynamic muscle training, relaxation training, or ordinary activity for chronic neck pain: randomised controlled trial. BMJ 2003;327:475.

[104] Pettersen V, Westgaard RH. Muscle activity in the classical singer's shoulder and neck region. Logoped Phoniatr Vocol 2002;27(4):169–178.

[105] Toivanen H, Helin P, Hanninen O. Impact of regular relaxation training and psychosocial working factors on neck–shoulder tension and absenteeism in hospital cleaners. J Occup Med 1993; 35(11):1123–1130.

[106] Holtermann A, Søgaard K, Christensen H, et al. The influence of biofeedback training on trapezius activity and rest during occupational computer work: a randomized controlled trial. Eur J Appl Physio 2008;104(6):983–989 Epub 2008 Aug 14.

[107] Little P. Randomised controlled trial of Alexander technique lessons, exercise, and massage (ATEAM) for chronic and recurrent back pain. BMJ 2008;337:a884.

[108] Fischer AA, Chang CH. Electomyographic evidence of paraspinal muscle spasm during sleep in patients with low-back pain. Clin J Pain 1985;1:147–154.

[109] Flor H, Furst M, Birbaumer N. Deficient discrimination of EMG levels and overestimation of perceived tension in chronic pain patients. Appl Psychophysiol Biofeedback 1999;24(1):55–66.

[110] Blanchard EB, Jurish SE, Andrasik F. The relationship between muscle discrimination ability and response to relaxation training in three kinds of headaches. Appl Psychophysiol Biofeedback 1981;6(4):537–545.

[111] Hamberg-van Reenen HHA. systematic review of the relation between physical capacity and future low back and neck/shoulder pain. Pain 2007; 130(1–2):93–107.

[112] Bronfort G, Evans R, Nelson B, et al. A randomized clinical trial of exercise and spinal manipulation for patients with chronic neck pain. Spine 2001;26(7):788–797.

[113] Ylinen J, Takala EP, Nykanen M, et al. Active neck muscle training in the treatment of chronic neck pain in women: a randomized controlled trial. JAMA 2003;289 (19):2509–2516.

[114] Waling K, Sundelin G, Ahlgren C, et al. Perceived pain before and after three exercise programs – a controlled clinical trial of women with work-related trapezius myalgia. Pain 2000;85(1–2):201–207.

[115] Waling K, Järvholm B, Sundelin G. Effects of training on female trapezius Myalgia: An intervention study with a 3-year follow-up period. Spine 2002; 27(8):789–796.

[116] Ahlgren C, Waling K, Kadi F, et al. Effects on physical

performance and pain from three dynamic training programs for women with work-related trapezius myalgia. J Rehabil Med 2001;33(4):162–169.

[117] Andersen LL, Andersen CH, Zebis MK, Nielsen PK, Søgaard K, Sjøgaard G. Effect of physical training on function of chronically painful muscles: A randomized controlled trial. J Appl Physiol 2008;105(6): 1796–1801 Epub 2008 Oct 23.

[118] O'Leary S, Falla D, Hodges PW, et al. Specific therapeutic exercise of the neck induces immediate local hypoalgesia. J Pain 2007;8(11):832–839 Epub 2007 Jul 19.

[119] Falla D, Jull G, Hodges P, et al. An endurance-strength training regime is effective in reducing myoelectric manifestations of cervical flexor muscle fatigue in females with chronic neck pain. Clin Neurophysiol 2006; 117(4):828–837.

[120] Falla D, Jull G, Hodges P. Training the cervical muscles with prescribed motor tasks does not change muscle activation during a functional activity. Man Ther 2008;13 (6):507–512 Epub 2007 Aug 27.

[121] van Tulder M, Malmivaara A, Esmail R, Koes B. Exercise therapy for low back pain: a systematic review within the framework of the Cochrane collaboration back review group. Spine 2000;25(21):2784–2796.

[122] Delcanho RE, Kim YJ, Clark GT. Haemodynamic changes induced by submaximal isometric contraction in painful and non-painful human masseter using near-infra-red spectroscopy. Arch Oral Biol 1996;41(6):585–596.

[123] Larsson SE, Larsson R, Zhang Q, et al. Effects of psychophysiological stress on trapezius muscles blood flow and electromyography during static load. Eur J Appl Physiol Occup Physiol 1995;71(6): 493–498.

[124] Maekawa K, Clarck GT, Kuboki T. Intramuscular hypofusion, adrenergic

receptors, and chronic muscle pain. J Pain 2002;3(4):251–260.

[125] Kadi F, Ahlgren C, Waling K, et al. The effects of different training programs on the trapezius muscle of women with work-related neck and shoulder myalgia. Acta Neuropathol 2000;100(3):253–258.

[126] Prior BM, Lloyd PG, Yang HT, et al. Exercise-induced vascular remodeling. Exerc Sport Sci Rev 2003;31(1):26–33.

[127] Soares JM. Effects of training on muscle capillary pattern: intermittent vs continuous exercise. J Sports Med Phys Fitness 1992;32(2):123–127.

[128] Soares T, Knutsson A, Puntschart A, et al. Increased expression of vascular endothelial growth factor in human skeletal muscle in response to short-term one-legged exercise training. Pflugers Archiv 2002;444(6):752–759.

[129] Sjölander P, Michaelson P, Jaric S, et al. Sensorimotor disturbances in chronic neck pain range of motion, peak velocity, smoothness of movement, and repositioning acuity. Man Ther 2008; 13(2):122–131.

Neuromuscular considerations in managing individuals with central nervous system damage

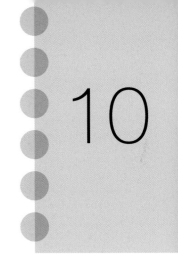

10

A young teenager with cerebellum tumour, with loss of coordination and balance, a young sports person with partial cervical cord damage with complex movement control losses, a stroke patient who has little use of one side of the body. These patients are presenting with extensive and diverse motor losses. How can neuromuscular rehabilitation help and how would the management differ between the conditions? Would it be different from neuromuscular rehabilitation of musculoskeletal injuries?

From a movement-control perspective the main difference between patients with intact and with damaged central nervous systems (CNS) lies in the magnitude of motor losses and the potential for recovery. Central damage is associated with more extensive motor control losses, longer rehabilitation duration and, frequently, only partial recovery.[1] However, the underlying principles of rehabilitation remain unchanged: the use of a functional approach in rehabilitation, the use of skill and ability-level rehabilitation and applying the principles of motor adaptation (Table 10.1).

The motor process in central injury

From a functional perspective CNS damage can be viewed as a processing failure and miscommunication within the motor system (Fig. 10.1). It is the incomplete and fragmented progress of the motor process from one stage to another: the organizer of movement has become partly disorganized.

Damage to the higher centres may impede the individual's ability to perceive incoming information, analyse it, integrate the information into movement strategies and carry out a skilful action.[2] Furthermore, under normal circumstance the spinal motor centres are under the dominant and integrative influence of the higher motor centres. Following damage to the higher centres, activity in the spinal motor centres may become disorganized, resulting in dysfunctional muscle recruitment and reflexes (Fig. 10.1).

Abilities affected

Central damage can result in complex and widely varying movement control losses. A description of all the potential damage and related functional changes is outside the scope of this book. However, the observable control changes can be analysed using the motor complexity model (Ch. 3).

In CNS damage there will be direct control losses in composite abilities, as well as synergistic and parametric abilities (Fig. 10.2).[3] In central damage the change in abilities represents real losses, whereas in the intact system, such as in musculoskeletal injuries, the change in abilities is mostly a strategic reorganization of movement. Hence, central damage is more difficult to recover than adaptive reorganization.

Within the parametric abilities, force control is commonly affected, with either loss (hypotonic) or abnormal increase in involuntary force seen as hypertonicity.[4–7] Some patients may find it difficult to "turn the muscle off," which also represents loss of force control (Ch. 3). Interestingly,

Table 10.1 Difference and similarity in neuromuscular rehabilitation for individuals with intact and damaged central nervous system

Factors in neuromuscular rehabilitation	Central nervous system	
	Intact	**Damaged**
Functional approach	Easily applied for most conditions	Use what the patient already knows May have to use extra-functional for those with severe motor losses
Cognitive	Cognitive elements easily applied Use external focus	May suffer from cognitive losses, which would impede motor recovery May need to revert to internal focus and use motor imagery
Being active	Engages the full motor process	As in intact In complete loss of voluntary movement the patient may need passive movement
Feedback	Acuity changes, often minor Feedback using verbal visual and manual guidance	True proprioceptive loss Feedback same as in intact, but therapist may need to stimulate proprioception by passive movement if patient unable to move
Repetition	Varied practice with random mix of tasks	May benefit from tasks that are practised individually, repetitively and with little variation
Similarity	Keep it similar to functional movement	As in intact. In severe losses, where functional movement is not possible may have to use extra-functional movement
Recovery duration	Weeks	Months to years
Recovery success	Mostly full	Partial

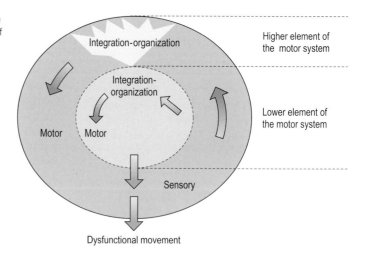

Fig. 10.1 • In central nervous system damage there is interruption to the normal organization of motor processes. Under these circumstances, the lower more reflexive elements of the motor system may become more dominant.

when a stroke patient is taught how to relax the forceful reflexive hypertonic muscle, a weak voluntary force ability is often found to be underlying it.[8] Velocity is often affected, with the patient only able to produce slow movements in a limb or during more general patterns such as walking.[9,10] A change in velocity control may also manifest as a sudden loss of control at certain angles within a movement range. For example, a stroke patient may be able to move the knee into

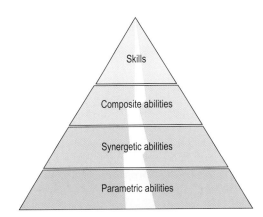

Fig. 10.2 • In central damage it is likely that most motor abilities will be affected.

extension while maintaining a constant velocity; at a certain angle the movement will be taken over by a fast reflexive extension. Length control often manifests as chronic dysfunctional shortening of the hypertonic muscles.[11]

Various factors within movement synergism are likely to be affected by central damage. It will include failure relative force, velocity and length, timing and duration of muscle activation,[12] or the dominance of one of the synergistic patterns.[13] For example, the hypertonicity and rigidity during movement can be seen as uncontrolled co-contraction.[13,14] Dynamic co-contraction loss can be seen in patients who can control movement in one plane, as long as they are supported bilaterally. Joint flexion contractures can be viewed as the dominance of one group of muscles over its synergistic group.[9] Loss of rhythmic movement such as arm swing can be viewed as loss of reciprocal activation.

The composite abilities can be affected either directly or due to the knock-on effect from parametric and synergistic ability losses. This would include losses to all coordination levels.[11,15] Loss of fine control can often be seen as the inability to manipulate objects with the hand.[16] Single-limb coordination loss is often evident as the inability to control the movement at a specific joint, or to integrate it with other joints into a synchronous limb movement.[17,18] Multi-limb coordination losses are often seen in activities such as rhythmic arm swinging during walking,[19] where each side can be swung separately but not together. Similarly whole-body dis-coordination is evident in loss of synchronization of the different body masses during movement.[10,20]

Relaxation ability is also important in rehabilitating movement control in patients with central damage. It is the flip side of motor activation: it requires motor control and, hence, may facilitate recommunication within the motor system; helping to re-establish central inhibitory influences. Basmajian[21] pointed out that patients with CNS damage can fully relax their hypertonic muscles to electromyogram (EMG) silence. A potent long-term control of hypertonicity could be to teach the patient focused motor relaxation of the affected muscles (Ch. 9). For example, in one particular stroke patient, the hand and wrist were locked solid into flexion contracture over a period of 5 years. Initially, the patient's partner would have to use all her strength to prise the hand open. Using focused motor relaxation, the patient learned to overcome this motor pattern and maintain the hand relatively relaxed and unclenched. This improvement remained unchanged and is maintained throughout the day and night (autonomous phase of learning).

Patients with central damage may present with a longer transition time when performing a variation within the same or between dissimilar tasks, e.g. the transition time to turning around during walking or from sitting to standing.[22]

Balance ability/postural stability is frequently affected in CNS damage.[23,24] It can arise from central balance losses or represent loss in other composite abilities, such as whole-body coordination or synergistic control in lower limb or trunk.[25]

The patient's clinical progress may not translate immediately into improvement in daily activities.[23] In order to perform a particular skill several underlying abilities need to recover to a certain critical level. A patient may have difficulties in raising their hand to the mouth, although the force and speed of arm movement may have improved. This could happen if there is a lag in improvement in other abilities, such as single-limb coordination or synergistic control at a specific joint.

Sensory-proprioceptive abilities

Proprioceptive losses are often varied and include a reduced perception of joint position and of movement, and an inability to feel muscle activity or to determine the force used. It will also affect the more complex sensory abilities such as limb/body orientation and composite sensory ability.

The proprioceptors are still "out there", but the centre cannot perceive them. This preservation of peripheral mechanisms of proprioception provides the potential for re-communication by the "rewiring" of alternative routes (Ch. 6).

Under normal circumstances the motor system is centrally controlled with proprioception providing feedback (Ch. 2). Following central damage, there is a loss of the dominant integrative influences from supraspinal centres. The consequence may be an increase in the influence that proprioceptors have over the lower spinal motor centres. Consequently, the segmental influence of the mechanoreceptors will become exaggerated, resulting in dysfunctional muscle activity and reflexes.[26] Such reflex responses seem to be more prominent during passive stimulation of the limb.[27] When the limb is actively used, these reflex influences tend to diminish,[27] probably due to the overriding influences of the higher centres. Hence, using active movement during rehabilitation may be more useful than trying to abolish the dysfunctional reflexes.

Neuromuscular rehabilitation in central nervous system damage

The aim in neuromuscular rehabilitation is to facilitate recovery by providing movement-related cognitive stimulation and physical challenges.[28,29] In response to such physical challenges the nervous system has been shown to undergo remarkable neural plasticity with related improvements in movement. This plasticity is marked by formation of new pathways by neuronal sprouting, formation of new synapses and the shifting of movement integration to non-affected parts of the brain (Ch. 6).[28-43]

The treatment programme consists of the three basic principles of neuromuscular rehabilitation: functional movement (using what the patient already knows), focus on skill/ability-level rehabilitation depending on the patient's capacity and facilitating more effective long-term neuromuscular recovery by the use adaptation code elements. Patients who have suffered substantial motor losses and who cannot perform any functional movement could be started on ability-level rehabilitation. Equally, rehabilitation should not regress to a level below the patient's movement capacity (Ch. 11).

Using the code for neuromuscular adaptation

Use of cognition

Cognitive abilities play an important part in the capacity to learn and recover functional movement in patients with CNS damage (Fig. 10.3).[2] Working in the cognitive dimension includes the use of attention and focus, and providing the patient (and their carers) with the understanding of the treatment goals and the principles used to achieve them. Patients who suffer cognitive losses may find it difficult to utilize these cognitive strategies and consequently a slower rate of recovery. Some of these cognitive abilities are described in Box 10.1.

Within the cognitive dimension internal and external focus is used pragmatically. The ideal is external focus on the goal of movement or overall task. This fits well with skill-level rehabilitation. However, some patients who have major movement losses may revert to using internal focus.

The ultimate aim of the treatment is to move from the cognitive to the autonomous/subconscious execution of movement. This can be achieved by adding simultaneous activities (multi-tasking) that require a different focus of attention.

Being active, feedback and repetition

The patient should be encouraged to actively perform the movement whenever possible. This will

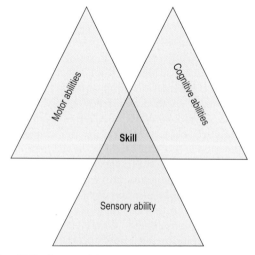

Fig. 10.3 • In central damage the skill of movement may be affected due to losses in cognitive, sensory and motor abilities.

Box 10.1

Cognitive abilities: the ability to perform a motor task is partly dependent on the cognitive abilities of the patient

- Attention or concentration
- Ability to initiate, organize or complete tasks
- Ability to sequence, generalize or plan
- Insight/consequential thinking
- Flexibility in thinking, reasoning, or problem-solving
- Judgment or perception
- Ability to acquire or retain new information
- Ability to process information

engage all the different motor stages (Ch. 2). Active movement is ideal, but if not possible, start with assisted passive movement. In hemiplegic stroke patients, passive movements elicited some of the brain patterns seen during active movements.[44]

Feedback can take several forms. It can be in the form of verbal or visual guidance, by demonstrating the movement. Manual guidance can be used to assist and correct movement pattern. Intrinsic feedback (proprioception) can be stimulated by passive movement, skin rubbing, firm holding and massaging. Several studies have demonstrated that such sensory stimulation can improve the sensory and motor ability of stroke patients.[45–47] However, passive forms of sensory stimulation are only likely to have a limited effect on motor learning/adaptation (Chs 2, 4 & 13). Proprioception may be enhanced by performing the movement with eyes shut. Conversely, vision can be used if proprioceptive loss is extensive.

In stroke patients repetition has been demonstrated to improve walking distance and speed, sit-to-stand tasks and the activities of daily living.[48] It was demonstrated that repetition can give positive gains in performance of a task even after one day of training.[49] On the first appointment I tell the patient and their carers to remember the three "Rs" – Repetition, Repetition and Repetition![50]

Similarity principle

The patient's own movement repertoire is used during the rehabilitation. This is in line with the functional approach similarity and context principles discussed in Chapter 5. If walking is being rehabilitated, then walking should be practised. If sitting to standing is being rehabilitated then this should be

practised, and so on. This is the message that has been repeated is recent systematic reviews.[51,52]

Underlying abilities should be challenged within functional movement. A reaching movement can be practised at different force levels, directions, speeds and repetitions (parametric abilities), using the full cycle of the paired movement, e.g. reaching and withdrawing the arm (synergistic ability). This movement should also be integrated into other composite abilities such as multi-limb coordination or organization rate. Coordination should be practised with movements that are similar to daily activities. This should include a mixture of single-limb, multi-limb and whole-body coordination practice.[53] Even balance ability should be practised in context. If walking balance is affected, balance should be practised in walking (dynamic balance) and not in standing (static balance). Standing balance may not transfer well to walking balance.[24]

When working with patients with low movement capacity rehabilitation might need to stray from the similarity principle. It may have to regress to ability-level rehabilitation on the treatment table or other body-support systems. However, the ultimate goal should be functional rehabilitation at skill level.

Summary points

- Many of the principles of neuromuscular rehabilitation can be applied during the management of individuals who suffer CNS damage.
- Both skill- and ability-level rehabilitation should be used simultaneously.
- The rehabilitation plan should contain the motor adaptation elements – cognition, active, feedback, repetition and similarity.
- Keep the training as close as possible to daily functional movement.
- Avoid complex movements that are not within the normal movement repertoire of the individual – train them in something they already know (but can't do).
- Neuromuscular rehabilitation in central system damage is a long-term process, psychologically and physically demanding for both the patient and the therapist. Make it fun, interesting and continuously challenging.
- There is nothing like one brain to stimulate another.

References

[1] Hendricks HT, van Limbeek J, Geurts AC, et al. Motor recovery after stroke: a systematic review of the literature. Arch Phys Med Rehabil 2002;83(11):1629–1637.

[2] McDowd JM, Filion DL, Pohl PS, et al. Attentional abilities and functional outcomes following stroke. J Gerontol B Psychol Sci Soc Sci 2003;58(1):P45–P53.

[3] Katz RT, Rymer WZ. Spastic hypertonia: mechanisms and measurement. Arch Phys Med Rehabil 1989;70(2):144–155.

[4] Horstman AM, Beltman MJ, Gerrits KH, Koppe P, Janssen P, Elich P, et al. Intrinsic muscle strength and voluntary activation of both lower limbs and functional performance after stroke. Clin Physiol Funct Imaging 2008;28(4):251–261.

[5] O'Dwyer NJ, Ada L, Neilson PD. Spasticity and muscle contracture following stroke. Brain 1996; 119(Part 5):1737–1749.

[6] Ada L, Canning CG, Low SL. Stroke patients have selective muscle weakness in shortened range. Brain 2003;126(Part 3):724–731.

[7] Newham DJ, Hsiao SF. Knee muscle isometric strength, voluntary activation and antagonist co-contraction in the first six months after stroke. Disabil Rehabil 2001; 23(9):379–786.

[8] Ross SA, Engsberg JR. Relation between spasticity and strength in individuals with spastic diplegic cerebral palsy. Develop Med Child Neurol 2002; 44(3):148–1457.

[9] Vattanasilp W, Ada L, Crosbie J. Contribution of thixotropy, spasticity, and contracture to ankle stiffness after stroke. J Neurol Neurosurg Psych 2000;69:34–39.

[10] Archambault P, Pigeon P, Feldman AG, et al. Recruitment and sequencing of different degrees of freedom during pointing movements involving the trunk in healthy and hemiparetic subjects. Exp Brain Res 1999; 126(1):55–67.

[11] Canning CG, Ada L, O'Dwyer NJ. Abnormal muscle activation characteristics associated with loss of dexterity after stroke. J Neurolog Sci 2000;176(1):45–56.

[12] Wenzelburger R. Hand coordination following capsular stroke. Brain 2005;128(Part 1): 64–74.

[13] Hidler JM, Carroll M, Federovich EH. Strength and coordination in the paretic leg of individuals following acute stroke. IEEE Trans Neural Syst Rehabil Eng 2007;15(4):526–534.

[14] Levin MF, Selles RW, Verheul MH, et al. Deficits in the coordination of agonist and antagonist muscles in stroke patients: implications for normal motor control. Brain Res 2000;853(2):352–369.

[15] Wu CY, Chou SH, Chen CL, et al. Kinematic analysis of a functional and sequential bimanual task in patients with left hemiparesis: intra-limb and interlimb coordination. Disabil Rehabil Nov 2008;26:1–9 [Epub ahead of print].

[16] Welmer AK, Holmqvist LW, Sommerfeld DK. Limited fine hand use after stroke and its association with other disabilities. J Rehabil Med 2008;40(8):603–608.

[17] Kautz SA, Patten C. Interlimb influences on paretic leg function in poststroke hemiparesis. J Neurophysiol 2005; 93(5):2460–2473.

[18] Cirstea MC, Levin MF. Compensatory strategies for reaching in stroke. Brain 2000;123(Part 5):940–953.

[19] Ustinova KI, Fung J, Levin MF. Disruption of bilateral temporal coordination during arm swinging in patients with hemiparesis. Exp Brain Res 2006;169 (2):194–207.

[20] Esparza DY, Archambault PS, Winstein CJ, et al. Hemispheric specialization in the co-ordination of arm and trunk movements during pointing in patients with unilateral brain damage. Exp Brain Res 2003;148(4):488–497.

[21] Basmajian JV. Muscles alive: their function revealed by electromyography. Baltimore: Williams & Wilkins; 1978.

[22] Flansbjer UB, Miller M, Downham D, et al. Progressive resistance training after stroke: effects on muscle strength, muscle tone, gait performance and perceived participation. J Rehabil Med 2008;40(1): 42–48.

[23] Gok H, Geler-Kulcu D, Alptekin N, et al. Efficacy of treatment with a kinaesthetic ability training device on balance and mobility after stroke: a randomized controlled study. Clin Rehabil 2008;22(10–11): 922–930.

[24] Genthon N, Rougier P, Gissot AS, et al. Contribution of each lower limb to upright standing in stroke patients. Stroke 2008;39(6):1793–1799.

[25] Verheyden G, Vereeck L, Truijen S, Troch M. Trunk performance after stroke and the relationship with balance, gait and functional ability. Clin Rehabil 2006;20(5):451–458.

[26] Dietz V. Spastic movement disorder. Spinal Cord 2000; 38(7):389–393.

[27] Ada L, Vattanasilp W, O'Dwyer NJ, et al. Does spasticity contribute to walking dysfunction after stroke? J Neurol Neurosurg Psychiatry 1998;64:628–635.

[28] Johansen-Berg H, Dawes H, Guy SM, Smith SM, Wade DT, Matthews PM. Correlation between motor improvements and altered fMRI activity after rehabilitative therapy. Brain 2002;125(Part 12):2731–2734.

[29] Johansen-Berg H. Structural plasticity: rewiring the brain. Curr Biol 2006;17:4.

[30] Schaechter JD, Kraft E, Hilliard TS, et al. Motor recovery and cortical reorganization after constraint-induced movement therapy in stroke patients: a preliminary study. Neurorehabil Neural Repair 2002;16(4): 326–338.

[31] Rowe LB, Frackowiak RSJ. The impact of brain imaging technology on our understanding of motor function and dysfunction. Curr Opin Neurobiol 1999;9(6):728–734.

[32] Brion JP, Demeurisse G, Capon A. Evidence of cortical reorganization in hemiparetic patients. Stroke 1989;20(8): 1079–1084.

[33] Cao Y, D'Olhaberriague L, Vikingstad EM, et al. Pilot study of functional MRI to assess cerebral activation of motor function after poststroke hemiparesis. Stroke 1998; 29(1):112–122.

[34] Cramer SC, Nelles G, Benson RR, et al. A functional MRI study of subjects recovered from hemiparetic stroke. Stroke 1997;28:2518–2527.

[35] Cramer SC, Finklestein SP, Schaechter JD, et al. Activation of distinct motor cortex regions during ipsilateral and contralateral finger movements. J Neurophysiol 1999;81:383–387.

[36] Johansen-Berg H. Motor physiology: a brain of two halves. Curr Biol 2003;13:R802–R804.

[37] de Bode S, Mathern GW, Bookheimer S, et al. Locomotor training remodels fMRI sensorimotor cortical activations in children after cerebral hemispherectomy. Neurorehabil Neural Repair 2007;21(6): 497–508.

[38] Ding Y, Li J, Clark J, et al. Synaptic plasticity in thalamic nuclei enhanced by motor skill training in rat with transient middle cerebral artery occlusion. Neurol Res 2003;25(2):189–194.

[39] Ding Q, Vaynman S, Akhavan M, et al. Insulin-like growth factor I interfaces with brain-derived

neurotrophic factor-mediated synaptic plasticity to modulate aspects of exercise-induced cognitive function. Neuroscience 2006;140(3):823–833.

[40] Black JE, Isaacs KR, Anderson BJ, et al. Learning causes synaptogenesis, whereas motor activity causes angiogenesis, in cerebellar cortex of adult rats. Proc Natl Acad Sci USA 1990; 87(14):5568–5572.

[41] Anderson BJ, Li X, Alcantara AA, et al. Glial hypertrophy is associated with synaptogenesis following motor-skill learning, but not with angiogenesis following exercise. Glia 1994; 11(1):73–80.

[42] Anderson BJ, Alcantara AA, Greenough WT. Motor-skill learning: changes in synaptic organization of the rat cerebellar cortex. Neurobiol Learn Mem 1996;66(2):221–229.

[43] Luft AR, Waller S, Forrester L, et al. Lesion location alters brain activation in chronically impaired stroke survivors. Neuroimag 2004;21(3):924–935.

[44] Nelles G, Spiekermann G, Jueptner M, et al. Reorganization of sensory and motor systems in hemiplegic stroke patients. A positron emission tomography study. Stroke 1999;30(8): 1510–1516.

[45] Cambier DC, De Corte E, Danneels LA, et al. Treating sensory impairments in the post-stroke upper limb with intermittent pneumatic compression. Results of a preliminary trial. Clin Rehabil 2003;17(1):14–20.

[46] Eckhouse Jr RH, Morash RP, Maulucci RA. Sensory feedback and the impaired motor system. J Med Sys 1990;14(3):93–105.

[47] Magnusson M, Johansson K, Johansson BB. Sensory stimulation promotes normalization of postural control after stroke. Stroke 1994;25(6): 1176–1180.

[48] French B, Thomas LH, Leathley MJ, Sutton CJ, et al. Repetitive task training for improving functional ability after stroke. Cochrane Database Syst Rev 2007;(4): CD006073.

[49] Platz T, Bock S, Prass K. Behaviour among motor stroke patients with good clinical recovery: does it indicate reduced automaticity? Can it be improved by unilateral or bilateral training? A kinematic motion analysis study. Neuropsychologia 2001; 39(7):687–698.

[50] Hesse S, Werner C. Poststroke motor dysfunction and spasticity: novel pharmacological and physical treatment strategies. CNS Drug Rev 2003;17(15): 1093–1107.

[51] Van Peppen RP, Kwakkel G, Wood-Dauphinee S, Hendriks HJ, Van der Wees PJ, Dekker J. The impact of physical therapy on functional outcomes after stroke: what's the evidence? Clin Rehabil 2004;18 (8);833–862.

[52] van de Port IG, Wood-Dauphinee S, Lindeman E, et al. Effects of exercise training programs on walking competency after stroke: a systematic review. Am J Phys Med Rehabil 2007; 86(11):935–951.

[53] McCombe Waller S, Liu W, Whitall J. Temporal and spatial control following bilateral versus unilateral training. Hum Mov Sci 2008;27(5):749–758.

Developing a rehabilitation programme

11

This chapter aims to provide a framework for neuromuscular rehabilitation using the principles of motor control and adaption.

We can learn about sensory-motor rehabilitation by observing what individuals naturally do when they attempt to recover their movement losses. Most frequently they tend to use a mixed strategy of re-abilitation within skill-level rehabilitation. For example, a person with a shoulder injury, after a short period of rest, will attempt to use their shoulder in what looks like a challenge to the movement parameters (parametric abilities). They will try to reach further (challenging length control), progressively lift heavier objects (challenging force control) and attempt to move faster to reach (challenging velocity control). They will tend to increase the number of repetitions of specific tasks or to sustain particular arm postures as a challenge to endurance. Within that behaviour, a person will often be aware of what is wrong with their movement and try to correct it (cognition & feedback). They will be actively seeking to improve it (being active), they will repeat the action numerous times (repetition), and these challenges will be performed within their daily routines (similarity and functional movement). This is nature's "gold standard" for self-recovery.

Neuromuscular rehabilitation follows the same strategy. It uses three key principles:

1. Use of functional approach in rehabilitation
2. Use of skill/ability-level rehabilitation
3. Use of the code for neuromuscular adaptation.

The rehabilitation programme follows these principles using a threestep process. The first step is to identify activities from the patient's movement repertoire which will specifically challenge their control losses. The next step is prioritizing the level at which rehabilitation will be used (ability/skill levels). Within the ability level it includes identifying and challenging specific control losses/changes. Finally, the motor adaptation elements are incorporated into the overall management.

The recovery of motor control is an intrinsic person/body process. The role of neuromuscular rehabilitation is to create ideal conditions in which this process is optimized.

A functional approach

The aim of a functional approach in rehabilitation is to utilize movements that the patient already knows rather than teaching them something new (extra-functional, see Ch. 1). The challenges to the losses are selected from the patient's repertoire of general and special movement skills. This process of selection can be exemplified by the case study of a patient who had suffered acute peripheral nerve damage brought about by a disc prolapse. After spinal surgery she was left with a moderate foot drop. The special skills within her functional repertoire included performing music and treadmill running in the gym. The challenges for the leg and foot were selected from these movement experiences (Fig. 11.1). From the general skill level, the challenges included climbing stairs, two stairs at a time, walking on the heels or toes, balancing on the affected side, gentle forward lunges onto the affected foot or lunges initiated from the affected side. From the special-skill sphere, movements included foot tapping to music with the forefoot or heel (which she

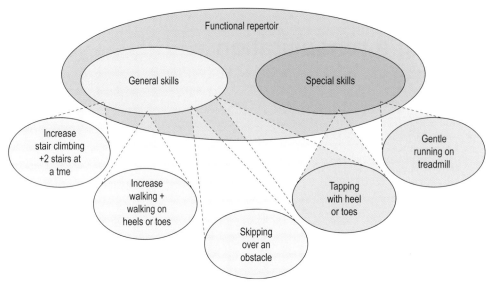

Fig. 11.1 • Movement challenges can be selected from the patient's own functional repertoire.

does all day), graded running on the treadmill in the gym and so on. The alternative would be to use extra-functional challenges (for her) such as introducing a wobble board, resistance bands or exercise machines at the gym, activities of which she has no experience. Is this approach more effective and one which she is more likely to adhere to (Ch. 1)?

Skill-level rehabilitation and re-abilitation

The next step in the rehabilitation process is to decide whether it should be at skill or ability level. Skill-level rehabilitation aims to engage the individual in executing their losses as closely as possible to the skills which have been affected. Ability-level rehabilitation (re-abilitation) aims to challenge specific losses in motor abilities (Fig. 11.2).

Skill-level rehabilitation assumes that by practising the affected movement/skill, the underlying motor "inabilities" will be challenged and, consequently, recover. Hence, for the patient described above much of the movement control of the leg and foot would be expected to recover by the time she returns to weight-bearing activities. These functional activities by themselves, and without further modification, will help to recover these particular movement losses.

However, some patients may present with persistent dysfunctional movement control, regardless of the fact that they are active (assuming that tissue

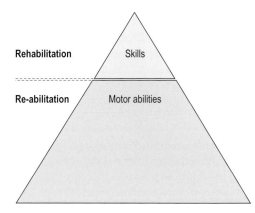

Fig. 11.2 • Rehabilitation can be at skill- or ability-level. Skill-level rehabilitation aims to restore movement losses by practising the movement affected. Ability-level rehabilitation (re-abilitation) focuses on challenging underlying motor-ability changes/losses.

repair processes have resolved). There could be several reasons for this:

1. Cognitive/psychological factors, injury beliefs and attitudes

2. Persistent pain or fears of it

3. Behavioural factors, such as task- or organizational-behaviour factors

4. Movement reorganization to injury ending up as an habitual movement pattern

5. Reorganization/change/losses in sensory-motor abilities.

Cognition about injury and pain, persistent pain and fear of it, behavioural factors and habitual patterns are all manageable within skill-level rehabilitation. In these conditions movement control is optimized by cognitive and behavioural means (Ch. 8) and there is no need to focus on specific motor losses.

There is also a possibility that imperfect practice leads to imperfect performance, i.e. when a patient is in pain they use, and inadvertently "learn", injury-related movement strategies. These patterns may persist even when the patients are no longer in pain. In this scenario, the rehabilitation is still at skill level, where the patient can be made aware of their movement "shortcomings". This is movement learning in a task-behaviour sphere and would be in the form of kinaesthetic feedback, providing information about the details and "correctness" of the movement ("hold the racket this way"), the movement sequences ("swing it like this") or the quality in performance ("good shot").

Another possibility is that certain underlying ability losses/changes maintain the movement dysfunction (motor inability). These inabilities could be residual elements of a control system that is still functioning in an injury mode (assuming there is no permanent and extensive tissue damage and the patient is not in severe pain). For example, the inability of a patient to execute a reaching movement (skill) may be due to local force or coordination losses in the arm (ability). A person with central nervous damage may be unable to walk normally (skill) due to losses associated with control of balance (ability).

In contrast to skill rehabilitation, at ability level, the challenges (training/practice/exercises) are specific to the underlying ability losses. In the case of balance, the therapist may challenge the patient's balance ability while standing or walking (Ch. 12). In the example of reaching, the underlying force or coordination abilities would be challenged during the reaching movement. In both of these examples the rehabilitation is challenging the particular inabilities within the skill level. This ensures that the treatment obeys, as closely as possible, the similarity and context principles.

It is not entirely clear why underlying inabilities do not spontaneously recover with normal functional movement. One likely possibility is that individuals may use movement strategies that circumvent and avoid an effective challenge of their motor losses. This may be observed in a person with balance inability. They may compensate for their losses by walking with a wider gait pattern, with shorter step intervals or shuffle along. They may simply avoid or minimize activities that are related to their loss. These patients would benefit from ability-level rehabilitation, as discussed above. In contrast, skill-level rehabilitation, which would encourage the patient to increase their walking distance, may not be effective in recovering balance ability. All that may happen is that patients will become very skilled at using the dysfunctional gait patterns.

In summary, the main difference between skill- and ability-level is that skill-level focuses on the correctness of movement or task. The patient is simply encouraged to carry out the movement that they are unable to perform. It may require some task-behaviour guidance but not special treatments or specific challenges that are beyond functional movement. Re-abilitation, on the other hand, requires more specialized, focused and specific challenges that target the underlying inabilities.

How to choose the level of rehabilitation

Generally, the treatments integrate skill- and ability-level rehabilitation, with the emphasis shifting between the two modalities.

Re-abilitation is rarely used outside the context of skill level. This would happen only for patients who have severe CNS damage, musculoskeletal injuries or post-surgery and who are unable to carry out any functional movement. For example, force re-abilitation may have to commence on the treatment table for a patient who cannot stand due to complete force losses in the leg. However, once the patient is able to weight-bear, the force re-abilitation should be in upright postures, i.e. re-abilitation within the context of a skill.

Merging the adaptive code with rehabilitation

The five elements of motor adaptation – cognition, being active, feedback, repetition and the similarity principle – should be integrated into both skill- and ability-level rehabilitation. Once a movement pattern/task has been identified as the goal of rehabilitation the patient should be made aware of its aims and focus on it (cognition). They will benefit from the therapist's guidance/aid (feedback). The movement should be repeated during and after the clinical session and resemble real functional patterns (repetition and similarity).

Similarity spheres

Similarity and context were identified as two of the key principles of motor adaptation (Ch. 5). They imply that effective rehabilitation is achieved when the training is similar to the goal task/skill. Perhaps it is important to examine what rehabilitation should be similar to. This depends on the functional repertoire of the person, the abilities affected, and which area of the body is the focus of treatment (Fig. 11.3). Hence, rehabilitation is often a combination of applying the similarity principle in these spheres:

- Skill
- Ability
- Functional characteristics of body area.

Skills can be divided into two broad areas. One comprises the *general skills* of doing everyday collective activities necessary for basic human needs (walk, stand, run, sit, dress, eat, etc.). The other comprises all the special activities that people undertake outside their daily actions, such as specialized occupational skills, sports, and physical hobbies (*special skills*).

Generally, treatment progresses from recovering the general skills to recovering the special skills. This sequence is used because the special skills often require a higher degree of motor control,

impose greater physiological and physical demands on the body and hence involve specific and more extended periods of rehabilitation. However, it does not exclude the possibility of starting at the special skill level if the general skills have recovered prior to rehabilitation.

These considerations will have an important bearing on the design of treatment. For example, leg rehabilitation of a tennis player and an office worker will share similarities in the general skill but different in the special skill spheres. An office worker may need leg rehabilitation that will promote normal functional daily use of the leg, i.e. walk, stand, etc. A tennis player would need a similar general skill rehabilitation as well as special skills rehabilitation. The challenges would include movements that resemble the actions of playing tennis such as jumping, lunging, sudden acceleration, sudden change of direction, explosive force, etc.

Another similarity consideration is which particular abilities have been affected. At ability level, treatment should seek to be specific to the underlying inabilities (see more below). As discussed elsewhere (Ch. 5), balance losses should be rehabilitated with balance challenge and force losses with force challenge. But balance cannot be rehabilitated by force, nor force by balance.

Also important within the similarity principle is which part of the body is rehabilitated. Clinically, the functional characteristics of the different body areas can be summarized into three broad groups: upper limb including hand, lower limb and trunk including head and neck. Obviously, arms don't do the actions that legs do. Therefore, leg rehabilitation is more about weight-bearing activities, such as balancing, walking, stepping, etc. Arm rehabilitation is more about reaching, holding, lifting, fine manipulation of objects, etc. Hence, knee rehabilitation is within the context of what a knee does, within the context of what a leg does, within the context of what the person does. This would be very different from shoulder rehabilitation, which would be executed within the context of what the person does with the arms.

This may seem like an obvious principle. However, often patients receive movement rehabilitation which is totally unrelated to the function of the particular part of the body. This includes floor exercise (core stability) for trunk rehabilitation, balancing exercise for the arm (using a Swiss ball), and lying, straight-leg rises to strengthen the leg muscle. All these rehabilitation regimes are totally dissimilar to the function and control of that particular body part.

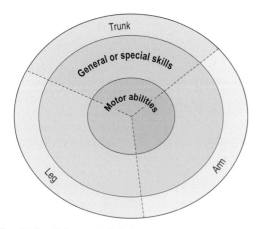

Fig. 11.3 • Spheres of similarity.

Table 11.1 The similarity grid

		Name the tasks affected:	Tick box
1. Body area	Arm		
	Trunk		
	Leg		
2. Ability	Parametric	Force	
		Velocity	
		Length	
		Endurance	
	Synergistic	Co-contraction (stability/steadiness)	
		Reciprocal activation (movement)	
	Composite	Coordination	
		Balance/postural stability	
		Transition rate	
		Relaxation	
3. Skill	General	List activities:	
	Special	List activities:	

In Table 11.1 the similarity grid is introduced as a clinical tool to help to develop the rehabilitation that is specific for their functional experience, remains close to the similarity principle and is specific to the control losses. It helps to identify the three areas of similarity that are particular to the individuals and their condition. The similarity grid should be used together with the history notes and clinical findings. It is a management and not a diagnostic tool. Copies of the similarity grid can be downloaded at www. cpdo.net/neuromuscularrehabillitation.

The similarity grid by an example

Let's look at the similarity grid using the patient with the foot drop as an example. The patient feels that the foot is weak and unsteady in all weight-bearing activities. Her sports activities are mainly running. How can we design the assessment and rehabilitation? Using the similarity grid we can start the process by testing the underlying parametric/synergistic abilities. It was identified that control of force, length, velocity and endurance has been affected (tick the appropriate boxes on the grid, Table 11.2A). This control loss is affecting the movement pairs in the foot (flexion–extension/inversion–eversion). This loss is present in static and dynamic of the foot, implying loss of control in the two synergistic patterns (tick "co-contraction" and "reciprocal activation" boxes). As a knock-on effect she has postural instability when attempting to stand on the affected leg (tick related box). Next on the grid is the body area in focus (tick "leg" box). Finally, the losses in the leg are influencing all the general and special skills such as running (tick related boxes). By observing the grid, the management and the type of challenges are mapped out clearly (see description at the beginning of this chapter).

Let us look at another example: the young tennis player who gradually developed knee pain due to dragging his leg on the ground when side-stepping (from Ch. 5). Examination of the limb revealed no motor losses. Tenderness was found on the medial aspect of the knee and it was diagnosed as a mild strain. The pain occurs only when he is playing tennis, so we can tick the "special skills" and the "leg" boxes (Table 11.2B). The fact that the onset of the condition was gradual implies that while playing he is habitually using a pattern that may stress the knee (rather than a traumatic injury). Hence, the management will be at skill-level focusing on the task-behaviour, correcting his side-step. Yes, it can be as simple as that. What is important here is that the grid is helping to prioritize the management but also suggesting what not to treat.

Another example is to look at the grid and the patient described in Chapter 10, who is suffering from chronic neck pain. Her conditions started gradually when she started a stressful computer-based job. She had no history of head/neck trauma. On examination, she had marked reduced neck rotation (Table, 11.2C, tick "length control") and loss of movement smoothness at the end ranges (tick "coordination" and "reciprocal activation"). We suspect from the history a loss of relaxation ability (tick box), which affects her throughout the day and during work (tick boxes). The management of this patient is described in Chapter 10.

Finally, in Table 11.2D is a description of a chronic stroke patient with mixed presentation on one side of the body: here all the boxes are ticked. This is to demonstrate the difference between managing a person with an intact and one with a damaged CNS. The general rule is that the more this grid fills up, the more extensive and complex is the patient's condition, often reflecting central damage.

Table 11.2 The use of the similarity grid for developing a treatment programme in different clinical presentations

Conditions:			A. Foot drop	B. Tennis player (medial knee pain)	C. Patient with chronic neck pain	D. Stroke patient (left side)
Name the tasks:			Weight-bearing	Playing tennis	Daily activities requiring neck movement	All activities
1. Body area	Arm					X
	Trunk				X (neck)	X
	Leg		X	X		X
2. Ability	Parametric	Force	X			X
		Velocity	X		X	X
		Length	X		X	X
		Endurance	X			X
	Synergistic	Co-contraction (stability/steadiness)	X			X
		Reciprocal activation (movement)	X		X	X
	Composite	Coordination			X	X
		Balance/postural stability	X			X
		Transition rate				X
		Relaxation			X	X
3. Skill	General	List activities:	X		X	X
	Special	List activities:	X	X	X	X

Context and specific injury rehabilitation (the amazing clinical shortcut)

Is motor rehabilitation of the spine different for a disc injury, degenerative changes of the facet joints or non-specific back pain? Is there a difference in neuromuscular rehabilitation of a patient with medial or lateral meniscus or cruciate ligament damage? Do we need intricate knowledge of all the motor changes associated with each condition in order to treat them effectively?

The answer is, probably not; which is very fortunate for all of us. This is largely due to the similarity principle. Ultimately, the body area in focus has to be rehabilitated similarly and in context to what it does functionally, regardless of the tissues involved (see similarity principle Ch. 5). Hence, neuromuscular rehabilitation of the back will be carried out in patterns that are similar to functional trunk movement during bending, lifting, pushing and standing, etc., regardless of which tissue is damaged. Knee rehabilitation will be in movement patterns that resemble knee movement during weight-bearing activities, again, regardless of the anatomical location of the injury.

The similarity principle provides us with a useful clinical short-cut: a context principle (Fig. 11.4). At the basic level of context, a joint does what a joint does. A hip, knee, ankle and foot all have their distinct physiological patterns of paired movements, such as flexion-extension, rotation etc. (*motion level*). At the next level of context all the leg joints move in patterns that reflect what the whole leg does (*context level*), within the next context level of what the person does with their legs, within their environment, e.g. stand, run, squat, climb stairs, etc.

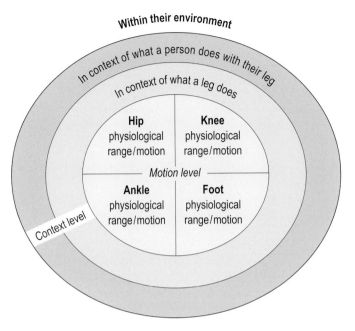

Within their environment

In context of what a person does with their leg

In context of what a leg does

| Hip physiological range/motion | Knee physiological range/motion |

Motion level

| Ankle physiological range/motion | Foot physiological range/motion |

Context level

Fig. 11.4 • The context principle applied to the lower limb. The inner circle represents the physiological range of a joint. Beyond that all other functions are within context (context level).

This means that at the lower level of context, which focuses on specific joints, the rehabilitation would be unique to each particular joint to account for their characteristic function. Hence, rehabilitation that commences on the treatment table will be markedly different from knee to the hip. However, once we move up one level, within the context of the whole leg, within the context of what a person does with it, the rehabilitation is no longer specific to a single joint. The leg will be rehabilitated as a whole in some functional pattern. It means that at this level hip, knee and ankle injuries are rehabilitated in much the same way, i.e. within weight-bearing activities (see part 2 video).

Rehabilitation and movement capacity

Ideally, a patient should be treated or trained at a level that matches or is somewhat above, their current movement capacity. If the patient can stand, rehabilitation of the leg should be in standing. Similarly, a patient who is suffering from lower back pain should be rehabilitated in upright tasks if they able to stand and move in upright posture. In these two clinical examples, there is no therapeutic/motor control value in challenging movement at a level below the patient's capacity. Exercising on the floor or treatment table would be below this capacity (which, unfortunately, is a very common approach for trunk rehabilitation in several physical therapies).

Is there a place for this capacity downgrading approach? It is reasoned that it is easier to train movement in a recumbent position and then transfer this experience to more complex upright tasks. Furthermore, it may help to reassure the patient that movement is safe. From motor learning and transfer perspective this is unlikely to be an effective training method (see similarity and context above). There may be some merit in a capacity-regressive rehabilitation as a way to reassure the patient that movement is OK. However, it can also convey the opposite message that movement is unsafe, especially if the patient is already able to perform some of their daily activities in upright postures.

Beyond the session: creating a challenging environment for repair and adaptation

Motor recovery is an adaptive and reparative process. It is dependent on the exposure of the individuals to the physical and cognitive-motor challenges that will drive this process.

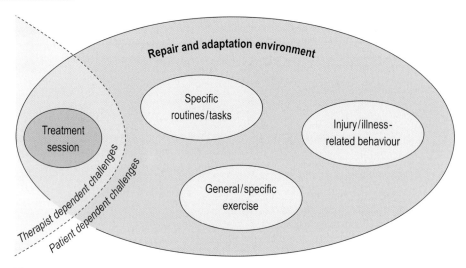

Fig. 11.5 • Co-creating a repair and adaptation environment to maintain the movement challenges throughout the day.

This can be achieved by co-creating with the patient an environment that challenges and competes with their current state. The re-created environment should extend to their daily activities. This can be achieved by using functional movement from the patient's daily routine or providing specific exercises that will challenge motor losses throughout the day (Fig. 11.5). This approach was exemplified in the management of the patient with the foot drop described above.

Rehabilitation that is limited to the clinic will occupy a small fraction of time within the patient's life and will, therefore, be less effective. The lack of challenges outside the session time will compete with the adaptation environment created during the session. The winner of this competition in adaptation will be the one the patient is most exposed to.

Summary points

- Recovery of motor control is an intrinsic person/nervous-system process.
- This recovery is dependent on psychological, behavioural, neurophysiological and tissue-related factors. Often many of these factors are interrelated.
- The role of neuromuscular rehabilitation is to optimize the recovery of movement control, working with all these factors.

- There are thee main principles to consider in neuromuscular rehabilitation: functional movement, skill- and ability-level rehabilitation, and the code for neuromuscular adaptation.
- A functional approach promotes the use of what the patient already knows. Challenges to specific motor losses can be found within the person's movement repertoire.
- At skill-level rehabilitation the patient simply aims to do the movements they can't do.
- Cognition about injury and pain, persistent pain and fear of it, and behavioural factors can all be managed within skill-level rehabilitation.
- Ability-level rehabilitation (re-abilitation) focuses on specific underlying motor losses that prevent the person from attaining their movement goals.
- The challenges to the motor abilities should be similar and within the context of functional activities.
- The challenges should be introduced at a level that matches, or is above, the patient's movement capacity.
- In the neurological dimension there is no injury-specific rehabilitation. An area is rehabilitated according to its function rather than to its underlying pathology.
- Rehabilitation is functional and like real-life movement. There is no need for fancy complicated stuff.

Motor abilities, assessment to challenge: re-abilitation

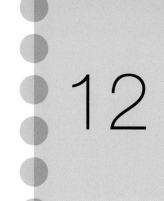

12

Within the motor complexity model the different motor abilities can be assessed, losses identified and recovered through specific movement challenges. The clinical process that focuses on these underlying control factors has been termed "re-abilitation".

Before describing the various assessments and challenges for the different abilities there are several clinical considerations related to re-abilitation:

- Assessment is a process of information gathering about the movement control of the individual. The aim of the assessment is to provide a better understanding of the patient's movement control rather than a diagnosis.
- Specific abilities can vary greatly between individuals or opposite sides of the body, even in normal healthy individuals. False positives are frequent and will contribute to clinical uncertainty. Several abilities should be assessed rather than relying on the outcome of a single assessments.
- Each motor ability can be assessed in several ways – there is no one single assessment procedure.
- In complex neuromuscular conditions, such as stroke, it may be difficult to assess all losses in one go. In these cases information is often gathered during several treatment sessions.
- Subjective responses from the patient are also important. During testing the therapist may not be aware of fine control failure. Yet the patient may report a subjective feeling of fatigue, weakness, an inability to control the movement or an inability to fully perceive the position of the limb.
- The assessments often become the challenge itself. This allows a smooth transition from

assessment to challenge without presenting the patient with an endless battery of tests.
- Often the challenge is characterized by introducing variations in the intensity, duration and repetition of particular movement patterns that enhance specific abilities.

The assessments and challenges of abilities described below are provided as examples (see summary, Table 12.1). Photographs of these challenges can be found on pages 142–161. The section containing the photographs is divided into challenges to control of the lower limb, upper limb and the trunk. A demonstration of these challenges (and much more) can be found in the accompanying DVD.

There is no strict protocol governing the assessment and challenge of abilities. Every patient and their condition is different. Furthermore, most conditions tend to vary and change over time. Be creative and invent assessments and challenges that suit the present clinical situation. There is no way to remember every single assessment – there are too many possibilities!

Parametric abilities: assessment and challenge

The four parametric abilities were identified as force, length, velocity and endurance abilities.

Force control

There are several factors that have to be considered when assessing and challenging force ability:

- Ability to fully relax
- Ability to produce maximal force

Table 12.1 Examples of assessments and challenges for the different motor abilities

Motor ability	Description	Assessment	Re-abilitation
		Parametric abilities	
Force Force relaxation Max force Force grading (dynamic or static)	The ability to provide adequate force for optimal execution of movement.	**Force relaxation:** Instruct patient to let go, assess the resistance to passive movement. **Maximal force:** Static force – patient holds a static position and resists therapist-imposed movement. Work within movement pairs (e.g. flexion–extension). Dynamic force – patient performs a cyclical task against resistance. **Force grading:** Patient gradually increases/decreases force against resistance.	**Force relaxation:** Patient has to make the limb heavy, instructed to perform movement with as little effort possible. Use contract–relax method. **Maximal force:** As assessment. Add different joint angles/limb position. **Force grading:** As assessment. Randomize the forces.
Length (also range or angle) Max length Max shortening Length grading	The ability to effectively regulate the range of movement.	**Max shortening and full length:** Compare passive active ranges of movement or active ranges of non-affected/affected sides. **Length grading:** Patient is instructed to slowly move the limb between two ranges. Look out for how smooth the movement is	As assessment. Change variables such as limb position, force (either dynamic or static) and velocity.
Velocity Max velocity Velocity grading	The ability to regulate the rate of movement.	**Max velocity:** Patient moves limb/trunk as fast as possible from one spatial position to another. **Velocity grading:** Movement at progressively increasing rate or alternating between fast and slow movement (tracking assessment).	As assessment. Change variables such as limb position by therapist moving hands apart to new positions.
Neuromuscular endurance	The ability to maintain a physical activity until it can no longer be continued.	How long a patient can perform a given task before fatigue sets in (dynamic endurance). How long a patient can maintain a particular position (static endurance). If in limbs, compare both sides.	As assessment.
Synergistic abilities			
Co-contraction Dynamic and static	The ability to control the active stability of joints.	**Static co-contraction:** Patient attempts to maintain a particular position against external perturbations. **Dynamic co-contraction:** Patient tries to maintain cyclical movement against sudden perpendicular perturbation by the therapist.	As assessment, but start low force and speed perturbations and gradually increase, as the patient is improving. Vary the joint position/plane of movement.

Reciprocal activation	The ability to control local movement at a joint.	Pendular movement of the limbs or trunk. Observe cyclical tasks.	As assessment. For cyclical tasks add parametric motor abilities: force, length, velocity and endurance. For challenging timing, instruct patient to perform low-velocity rhythmic cyclical movement. As their control improves increase the movement velocity.
Composite abilities			
Coordination	The harmonious and synchronous control of two or more joints or body masses.	Instruct the patient to perform different tasks, observe the ability to control the movement within the same limb and in relation to other limbs.	Encourage functional movement within single or multiple limbs. Vary limb positions, angles, force and velocity.
Balance and postural stability	The ability to maintain upright movement or stance efficiently and with minimal physical stress.	**Dynamic balance:** Observe tasks such as walking, walk and turn, hopping on single leg, etc. **Static balance:** Standing on both legs, narrow the standing base and finally single leg.	More of the assessment.
Transition time	The duration needed to re-organize movement between two dissimilar tasks and to carry out the subsequent task skillfully.	**Vertical transition:** Assess transition within the same ability by rapidly alternating between two extremes, e.g. fast-slow or forceful-gentle. **Lateral transition:** Take two abilities such as reciprocal activation and co-contraction and instruct the patient to change rapidly between them.	Same as assessment. Once specific contraction or composite abilities improve, introduce the transition rate by mixing the contraction abilities, e.g. moving at low force and fast, to suddenly shifting to a strong force and slow movement.
Motor relaxation	The ability to reduce neuromuscular activity to an optimal level necessary for maintaining a motor task or to become inactive.	Difficult to estimate during active movement. Sometimes postural indications, such as tensing the shoulders. Assess resistance to passive movement. Also palpate muscles during rest or during tasks (may not be very reliable assessment, consider adding contract–relax during the palpation).	Guide patient on how to relax while on the treatment table or during specific task, e.g. slowly turn your head while trying to make the neck soft.

• Ability to grade the movement force.

Assessing force control

Relaxation ability can be assessed by instructing the patient to let go and make the limb heavy. At this point the therapist moves the patient's limb passively while assessing the level of background resistance.

Resistance to passive movement of the neck and trunk/spine can be assessed more effectively when the patient is lying down. It assesses the resistance to movement between body masses rather than being a test for segmental or individual joint range of motion. For example, neck relaxation can be assessed by moving the head mass in counter-rotation to the thoracic mass.

Assessing muscle tension by palpation alone, although possible, can be misleading. This is partly because of the inaccuracy of palpation itself as a diagnostic tool,[1] but also due to the fact that passive resting muscle tone can be high, although the muscle is motorically silent.[2] One way to overcome this difficulty is to use contract–relax during palpation. The therapist can then compare the tightness (tone) in the muscle between the active and relaxed states.

Maximal force production can be assessed either in movement or in statically held positions. The test for control generally aims to encompass the movement pairs. For example, static force can be tested by instructing the patient to hold the limb in a particular position, say elbow flexed at 90 degrees. While in this position the force is challenged both in flexion and extension. Dynamic force can be assessed by instructing the patient to produce a repetitive reaching movement while providing resistance through the whole cycle of movement (challenging force within the synergistic pairs).

To test force grading control, simply ask the patient to perform the same movements but at different force levels, e.g. "try moving with the least amount of effort, try maximal effort and now try a force level in-between". Loss in control of force grading is more obvious in patients who had CNS trauma, but more difficult to assess in individuals with musculoskeletal injuries (who have an intact CNS).

Challenging force control

The challenge to force control is no different from the assessment; just do more of the same.

For motor relaxation, i.e. no force, the patient can be given instructions such as "make your limb heavy" or "imagine your muscles melting", etc. This approach is discussed in greater detail in Chapter 9 which examines non-traumatic pain conditions.

Maximal force can be challenged during movement or in held positions, as described in the test above. The movement patterns should be within normal functional arm movement, i.e. hand to mouth, tennis serve patterns, etc., continuously varying the angles and the forces applied. The patient is instructed to perform a movement such as reaching and retrieving, during which the therapist applies varying degrees of resistance (see Fig. 12.45).

The challenge of force can alternate between dynamic and static force. As the patient is moving their arm (dynamic) at different angles, instruct them to stop and hold that position (static). At that point the therapist applies force perturbation to the arm within the movement pairs (e.g. flexion-extension) or random challenges.

As discussed above, force grading challenge is more often used for patients with CNS damage. For example, to challenge force grading in the affected hand, the patient is instructed to hold and squeeze the therapist's hand. They are instructed to squeeze "hard", "soft" and in the "middle". They can also be instructed to gradually increase and decrease the force between these two extremes. As they improve, the instructions can become more random; "squeeze hard, medium, hard, soft, hard" and so on.

A note on force ability

Recent studies have demonstrated that functional weight-bearing exercises are as effective in improving force ability in the leg as specific knee-strengthening exercise.[3–5] However, the functional group benefited a bit more – there are added improvements in balance ability (146% improvement compared to only 34% in the strength group), and a tendency to equalize muscle strength imbalances between the dominant and non-dominant legs. Apart from these obvious advantages such functional challenges can be developed in clinic and as exercise without the need for any equipment (in my clinic I have only a treatment table and patients are given only functional exercise).

Another note on force, it has generally been assumed that fatigue and metabolite accumulation is a prerequisite for strength gains, i.e. pain = gain. However, a recent study has demonstrated subjects who weight-train with sufficient rest periods between sets have the same strength gains as subjects who train with fatigue.[3] This suggests that patients do not have to be put through a gruelling painful treatment to achieve force improvement (in particular if they are recovering from a painful condition).

Length control

There are several factors that have to be considered when assessing and challenging force ability:

- Full active range control
- Full active shortening control
- Grading of length.

Assessing length control

The full active range can be assessed by comparing it to the opposite side or to the passive range. Both length and shortening control should be examined when comparing the active-passive ranges of movement. Failure to actively reproduce the passive ranges may imply changes in length-shortening control of synergistic muscles. (Note: there is often a normal discrepancy between active and passive ranges, passive being greater than active range. Hence, in this assessment look out for gross differences).

Grading of length is usually a finer level of motor control. Hence, the loss of this control is more evident in individuals who have suffered CNS damage. For example, a stroke patient when instructed to gradually move the knee from flexion to extension may flick the knee into full extension, being unable to control the mid-ranges.

Challenging length control and functional stretching

An effective way to work on length control is to take the limb, trunk or neck passively to the end range. The patient is than encouraged to perform functional movements at the end range – *functional stretching* (see miscellaneous on DVD). For example, in the shoulder, fully flex the patient's shoulder passively (see Fig. 12.47). Once the full range is achieved, instruct the patient to perform any functional movement, such as waving or pulling and pushing a sash window. The advantage in this approach is that both sides of the movement pairs are being retrained simultaneously – the shortening control of shoulder flexors and lengthening control

of shoulder extensors (see also stretching versus length control, Ch. 3).

Velocity/speed control

The most common issues in velocity control are:

- Max velocity
- Ability to grade acceleration/deceleration.

Assessing velocity/speed control

An example of an assessment for this ability is to instruct the patient to move, as fast as possible, the affected limb between two positions marked by the therapist's hands (see Fig. 12.46). Another speed assessment is to observe the time a patient may need to complete a simple task such as getting up from sitting, walking a certain distance or the number of repetitions that can be achieved within a given time.

Somewhat different from speed of movement is the ability to grade the speed of movement. One way to test this ability is to instruct the patient to hold their arm, touching the therapist's hand. The therapist moves their hand in space at varying speeds while the patient attempts to track the therapist's hand movements.

Challenging velocity/speed control

Re-abilitation of velocity control is the same as the assessment. The patient is instructed to move their limb between the two spatial positions marked by the therapist's outstretched hands. Further challenge can be introduced by the therapist holding their apart in various positions - wider apart or in different planes of movement (see Fig. 12.46).

Endurance (neuromuscular)

Assessing endurance

Generally, endurance can be assessed by instructing the patients to perform repetitively specific tasks and looking for signs of fatigue (a gradual increase in pain and failure in voluntary activation).

The assessment of endurance can be by observing the patient perform repetitions of functional tasks such as walking, getting up from sitting, etc. It can also assess local fatigue in a limb. This type of assessment can be performed either in dynamic or static states of the limb. For example, endurance during dynamic conditions can be assessed by instructing the patient to move their limb repetitively between two positions and note how rapidly they fatigue.[6]

Static endurance can be assessed by instructing the patient to maintain a particular limb position, during which time the therapist applies force perturbations repetitively, in one or several directions.

Challenging endurance

Treatment is the same as the assessment. The challenge of endurance can be alternated between dynamic and static endurance.

> ### Clinical note
>
> Often training involves repetition to the point of fatigue; this is believed to be a signal for muscle adaptation or even motor learning. Although repetition is an important element for neuromuscular adaptation, fatigue is not.[3] If the patient fatigues too rapidly, they may be unable to carry out sufficient number of repetitions. This is important in situations where the re-abilitation is focused on abilities other than endurance or force, such as coordination, velocity and control of timing and duration of synergists.

Sometimes fatigue is the first or most obvious symptom of an underlying motor problem. For example, I am currently working with a patient who experiences disabling fatigue of the shoulder during swimming. He seems to have no other motor losses to the shoulder. Focusing on endurance ability has resulted in tripling his swimming distance.

Integrating parametric and synergistic abilities

The assessments and challenges of motor abilities are for movement control rather than for the assessment of individual muscles. As was discussed previously, muscles don't work alone but in complex synergisms (Ch. 3). It would be expected that muscle injury will result in control changes to the damaged muscle as well as all its synergists. For example, a biceps muscle injury is likely to influence the parametric control to biceps as well as all its synergists in the shoulder and elbow. Hence, the parametric abilities should be seen and challenged within the context of synergism and movement pairs (e.g. flexion/extension, Fig. 12.1).

Synergistic control

In the section above, some ideas were put forward for assessing and challenging the parametric abilities within their movement pairs/synergies. Unique to this level of motor control are the timing and duration of activation between muscle groups (or movement pairs).

Another consideration is the ability to utilize the correct pattern of synergism for particular movement requirements.

Fig. 12.1 • Parametric abilities should be integrated into the synergistic level, working in paired movement patterns. Avoid movements in a single direction and targeting single muscle groups.

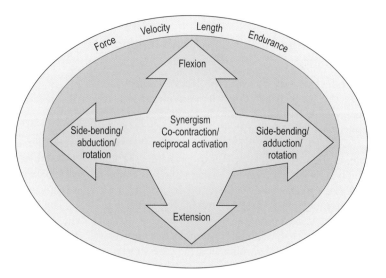

Synergistic abilities

Co-contraction assessment

Within co-contraction there are two patterns that can be assessed:

- Static co-contraction
- Dynamic co-contraction.

To assess static co-contraction, the patient holds the limb in the position to which the challenge is to be introduced. The therapist applies perturbations attempting to move the limb/trunk away from that position. These are low force and amplitude perturbations, applied rapidly with sudden changes in the direction of movement, usually within the movement pairs, e.g. flexion–extension (see Fig. 12.46). The different movement pairs can be challenged individually, in sequence or randomly.

When co-contraction is affected the patient will be unable to "stiffen" the joint to provide adequate resistance to the imposed movements. There is a perceivable delay before the patient is able to "kick-in" with a muscle contraction to resist the perturbation; particularly during the sudden change in direction. Another common observation is that patients with synergistic control losses may attempt to increase the force of co-contraction to overcome losses in timing.

This assessment should commence at a low perturbations rate and force, gradually increasing it as the patient becomes familiar with the movement.

This test can be repeated in different joint angles and ideally in positions where failure may be suspected. For example, instability may be more evident in plantar- rather than dorsi-flexion, a position where the foot is more likely to "twist" during weight-bearing activities.

To assess dynamic co-contraction, the patient can be instructed to move their limb in one plane, say, a sawing movement with their arm. As the patient is performing the task, the therapist introduces sudden unexpected perturbations perpendicular to the direction of movement (see Fig. 12.46). If the patient has good control over this ability they should be able to successfully maintain the movement in one plane.

Challenging co-contraction

Static co-contraction challenge is an extension of the assessment described above. The assessment then becomes the challenge by introducing the repetition element and varying the movement parameters (force, velocity length/angle).

Dynamic co-contraction re-abilitation can have two forms. One form is as described in the test above, where the patient tries to maintain movement in one plane against sudden perturbations. Another form utlizes the phenomenon that dynamic co-contraction is more evident during fine or fast movements (Ch. 3). Hence dynamic co-contraction can be challenged by introducing fast limb or trunk movements within a narrow range. The range can be determined by the therapist's hands. The patient is instructed to swing their limb or their trunk between these markers as fast as possible (same procedure as for reciprocal activation but faster, see Figs 12.46 & 12.61).

> ## Clinical note
>
> There are several conditions where dysfunctional co-contraction patterns are present (reflected in timing and duration changes).[7–14] This is often seen in psychomotor problems such as muscle tensing associated with stress or in patients with CNS damage (Chs 9 & 10). In these conditions the aim is to normalize co-contraction and allow more effective reciprocal activation. This can be achieved by guiding the patient on how to relax antagonistic muscle groups during movement. (It has been demonstrated that in some patterns of movement, co-activation virtually disappears when subjects are instructed to relax at the initiation of movement).[15] The re-abilitation goal is that movement which is dominated by co-activation will shift towards reciprocal activation with practice (see more in Ch. 3).[16]

Reciprocal activation assessment

The timing of reciprocal activation is very difficult to assess in clinic. The assessment is more observational, examining the "smoothness" or quality of movement. One method of examination is to instruct the patient to perform rhythmic pendular movement of the limbs or trunk (see Figs 12.19, 12.46 & 12.61). Pendular movements are predominantly reciprocal activation recruitments that involve rapid, out-of-phase, contraction and relaxation of the movement pairs. They are, therefore, useful to assess as well as challenge reciprocal activation ability.

Challenging reciprocal activation

Any cyclical and rhythmic movement will promote reciprocal activation of the synergists. Often the inability of the patient to produce smooth reciprocal movement is due to an uncontrollable and overriding co-contraction. Sometimes this can be reduced by simply instructing the patient to relax during the movement of the limb. Control of reciprocal activation may also be influenced by the velocity of movement. The challenge can start with slow reciprocal movements, during which the patient is instructed to make it "as smooth as possible", increasing the movement velocity as they improve.

Composite abilities

In Chapter 3 the composite abilities were identified as:

* Coordination
* Balance/postural stability
* Transition time
* Relaxation.

Coordination

There is no single way to assess coordination. Many of the tests are worked out on the spot depending on the area of the body affected. There are several coordination levels: fine control, single-, multi-limb and body coordination.

Coordination assessment

A simple way to assess coordination is to observe the quality of movement during particular tasks. Failure in coordination often manifests as the loss of smooth synchronized movement and an inability to accurately reach a target. Sometime losses in coordination are overcome by the patient reducing their movement velocity. The challenge to coordination can be made progressively more demanding by increasing the rate or the complexity of movement.

Upper limb (as an example)

Fine control in the hand can be assessed by instructing the patient to approximate the thumb and the fingers in different sequences, manipulate an object such as a pen between the fingers, or to simply write numbers or join dots on paper.

Single-limb coordination can be assessed by instructing the patient to alternately touch with their index finger two reference points, such as their other hand and the therapist's hand. To increase the challenge, this assessment can be performed at a progressively faster rate or by continuously changing the reference points. This is done by the therapist's moving their hand to different spatial positions. Another simple test is for the patient to touch and follow the therapist's hand as it is moving in space (see Figs 12.20 leg and 12.54 trunk; for arm see DVD).

Multi-limb coordination tests essentially examine the patient's ability to use the arms simultaneously and synchronously during specific tasks. It can start as a simple test to see if the patient can swing their arms as if walking, passing an object between the hands to more demanding tests such as tracking with both arms the movements of the therapist's hands.

Whole body coordination can be assessed by observing the patient performing whole body daily tasks such as walking into the room, getting up from sitting, dressing, etc.

Challenging coordination

Re-abilitation of coordination at all levels is the same as the assessments described above.

Balance and postural instability

Balance assessment

Balance should be tested both while standing (static) and during movement (dynamic).

Static balance can be assessed by progressively narrowing the standing base in order to increase the demand on balance control; starting with feet apart, side-by-side, one foot directly in front of the other and eventually standing on one leg. Further balance challenges can be achieved by balancing on the ball of the feet, closing the eyes or drawing an imaginary number with the non-weight-bearing leg (see Figs 12.36–12.39). In this assessment, look out for the time spent on one leg, and how demanding the balance for the weight-bearing foot is. Fine-balance deficit may only become apparent as the base becomes smaller and vision is reduced.[17]

Dynamic balance assessment can take several forms. The most immediate is to observe the patient perform activities such as walking across the room, walking around the table, climbing stairs, etc. There are several indicators when dynamic balance is affected such as use of broader walking base, the time spent on the affected side (shorter duration), a shuffled walk (not raising the feet to clear the ground), taking small steps and unusual body sway (some of these findings may also represent other motor control losses).

The single leg balance described above also can be turned into a dynamic assessment by instructing the patient to hop on one leg. Forward-backward, side-to-side and diagonal skipping can be added to further challenge dynamic control.

Most of the tests described above for balance are initiated and performed by the patient. As such this challenge is *expected* and the patient has sufficient time to organize for it (in anticipated tasks there is motor organization before the movement commences, a "feed-forward" phenomenon). However, in real life situations there are *unexpected* events that challenge balance, such as tripping or being jostled by others. Often, patients with balance deficits may find it difficult to meet such challenges since there is no anticipatory postural adjustment. The patient has, therefore, to rely on their transition time (which is a mixture of reaction and movement time).

Unexpected challenges that resemble real life situations can be introduced during the balance tasks. The therapist can stand behind the patient and introduce small amplitude perturbations (pushes) in different directions. These challenges can be introduced during static balance or during walking; in particular during the stance phase of the gait cycle of the affected limb (see Fig. 12.38).

Patients who have central balance losses can also be assessed in unsupported sitting.[18] When gently jostled there may be a small but observable delay before they are able to correct their sitting position. I have occasionally observed this in elderly patients suffering with mild CNS degeneration. This sometimes can help to differentiate problems of motor loss affecting the legs from those that are centrally mediated.

Challenging balance/postural instability

Challenging balance is an extension of the assessments.

Transition time

Transition time is the ability to rapidly and smoothly organize movement from one particular action to another. This can be within a single ability (*vertical transition time*), such as alternating between fast and slow movements or between any two abilities or tasks (*lateral transition time*). This can be assessed by introducing sudden, unexpected changes to the movement.

Transition time assessment

A vertical assessment of transition can be the observation of the patient's capacity to perform two extremes of a single ability. For example in force control, to quickly alternate between full relaxation and maximal contraction, in speed control the capacity to alternatively produce slow and fast movements, such as in the arm tracking challenge.

Transition time can be also assessed by introducing sudden changes in the direction and range. For example, in the test where the patient has to move their arm between two spatial positions (see above speed ability), the therapist can introduce sudden changes in the distance between, or the position of, the two hands.

Transition time assessment in balance ability could be to alternate between dynamic and static balance, for example quickly walk then suddenly stopping and balancing on a single leg.

Transition time can be assessed by instructing the patient to perform two different tasks, such as observing the time it take sitting to standing, etc. (it also requires other abilities such as speed of movement). It can also be assessed by instructing the patient to alternate between two abilities, such as reciprocal activation and co-contraction. For example, the patient could start by tracking with their arm the therapist's hand. At particular positions the therapist suddenly stops and the patient has to maintain that position while the therapist applies the co-contraction challenge described above. Failure often manifests as a delay in organizing the stiffness (co-contraction) needed to overcome the perturbations.

Occasionally it may be possible to estimate reaction time. For example the patient, while sitting on the treatment table, is instructed to maintain their knee flexed at 90 degrees. The therapist applies a force to flex the knee against the patient's resistance. The therapist suddenly removes their hand but the patient has to maintain the knee position (at 90 degrees, without overshooting into extension). The extent to which the patient can maintain the original flexed position provides a rough estimate of the reaction time.

A variation of the reaction time element is to instruct the patient to simultaneously tap both their hands on the therapist's hands. The therapist surprises the patient by continuously changing the position of the hands, which the patient is trying to follow. How well the patient is able to follow the sudden change of position can provide some assessment of their reaction time.

Challenging transition time

The challenges are an extension of the assessment described above.

Vertical and lateral transitions are often mixed during the re-abilitation. This can be exemplified in treating the hand of a CNS-damage patient. At first, work with each contraction ability separately (vertical transition); moving the thumb at different speeds, and forces. Once these specific abilities improve, introduce the lateral transition rate by mixing the contraction abilities, e.g. instructing the patient to move the thumb slowly and fast, to suddenly shifting to a strong force and slow movement, etc.

Motor relaxation

Psychomotor relaxation assessment and challenge

This ability can be difficult to fully assess. Often the diagnosis is made from the case history,

particularly in pain conditions where there is no history of physical trauma. Otherwise the assessment and challenge of this ability is similar to those described for force relaxation ability described above. Motor relaxation training was discussed in Chapter 9. For discussion on differences between force relaxation and motor relaxation see Chapter 3.

Summary points

- Re-abilitation is the process of assessing and challenging specific motor abilities.
- The aim of the assessment is to provide a better understanding of the patient's motor abilities. It is a process of information gathering.
- Specific abilities can vary greatly between individuals or opposite sides of the body, even in normal healthy individuals.
- Abilities can be assessed in many different ways.
- Many of the assessments often become the challenge itself.
- The challenge is often characterized by introducing variations in the intensity extent (length), duration and repetition of particular movement patterns.
- There is no strict protocol for re-abilitation. Be creative and invent assessments and challenges that suit the situation.

References

[1] Stochkendahl MJ, Christensen HW, Hartvigsen J, et al. Manual examination of the spine: a systematic critical literature review of reproducibility. J Manipulative Physiol Ther 2006;29(6): 475–485 485.e1–485.e10. Review.

[2] Lederman E. The science and practice of manual therapy. Edinburgh: Elsevier; 2005. p. 197–201.

[3] Folland JP, Irish CS, Roberts JC, et al. Fatigue is not a necessary stimulus for strength gains during resistance training. Br J Sports Med 2002;36(5):370–373.

[4] Beutler AI, Cooper LW, Kirkendall DT, et al. Electromyographic analysis of

single-leg, closed chain exercises: implications for rehabilitation after anterior cruciate ligament reconstruction. J Athl Train 2002;37(1):13–18.

[5] Liu-Ambrose T, Taunton JE, MacIntyre D, et al. The effects of proprioceptive or strength training on the neuromuscular function of the ACL reconstructed knee: a randomized clinical trial. Scand J Med Sci Sport 2003;13(2):115–123.

[6] Rosendale L, Larsson B, KristiansenJ , et al. Increase in muscle nociceptive substances and anaerobic metabolism in patients with trapezius myalgia: microdialysis in rest and during exercise. Pain 2004;112:324–334.

[7] Levin MF, Dimov M. Spatial zones for muscle coactivation and the control of postural stability. Brain Res 1997;757(1):43–59.

[8] Levin MF, Selles RW, Verheul MH, Meijer OG. Deficits in the coordination of agonist and antagonist muscles in stroke patients: implications for normal motor control. Brain Res 2000;853(2):352–369.

[9] Tedroff K, Knutson LM, Soderberg GL. Synergistic muscle activation during maximum voluntary contractions in children with and without spastic cerebral palsy. Dev Med Child Neurol 2006;48(10):789–796.

[10] Farmer SF, Sheean GL, Mayston MJ, et al. Abnormal motor unit synchronization of

antagonist muscles underlies pathological co-contraction in upper limb dystonia. Brain 1998;121(Part 5):801–814.

[11] Preibisch C, Berg D, Hofmann E, et al. Cerebral activation patterns in patients with writer's cramp: a functional magnetic resonance imaging study. J Neurol 2001; 248(1):10–17.

[12] Hughes M, McLellan DL. Increased co-activation of the upper limb muscles in writer's cramp. J Neurol Neurosurg Psychiatry 1985;48(8):782–787.

[13] Fernández-de-Las-Peñas C, Falla D, Arendt-Nielsen L, et al. Cervical muscle co-activation in isometric contractions is enhanced in chronic tension-type headache patients. Cephalalgia 2008;28(7):744–751. Epub 2008 May 5.

[14] Oksanen A, Pöyhönen T, Ylinen JJ. Force production and EMG activity of neck muscles in adolescent headache. Disabil Rehabil 2008;30(3):231–239.

[15] Yamazaki Y, Ohkuwa T, Suzuki M. Reciprocal activation and coactivation in antagonistic muscle during rapid goal-directed movement. Brain Res Bull 1994;34(6):587–593.

[16] Psek JA, Cafarelli E. Behavior of coactive muscles during fatigue. J Appl Physiol 1993; 74(1):170–175.

[17] O'Connell M, George K, Stock D. Postural sway and balance testing: a comparison of normal and anterior cruciate ligament deficient knees. Gait Posture 1998;8(2): 136–142.

[18] Verheyden G, Nieuwboer A, De Wit L, et al. Trunk performance after stroke: an eye catching predictor of functional outcome. J Neurol Neurosurg Psychiatry 2007;78(7):694–698.

Demonstration of challenges

Index of Figures 12.2–12.64				
Abilities		**Leg/hip**	**Arm/shoulder**	**Trunk/spine**
Co-contraction	Force Velocity Length/ range	Figs 12.2–12.11 (non-context, pp. 142–144) Figs 12.21–12.25 (in context, pp. 149–150)	Figs 12.40–12.44 (pp. 157–158)	Figs 12.48–12.51 (non-context, pp. 160) Figs 12.55–12.60 (in context, pp. 163–164)
Reciprocal activation	Force Velocity Length/ range	Figs 12.12–12.19 (non-context, pp. 145–148) Figs 12.26–12.34 (in context, pp. 151–153)	Figs 12.45–12.47 (pp. 159)	Figs 12.52–12.53 (non-context, pp. 161) Figs 12.61–12.64 (in context, pp. 165–166)
Coordination		Figs 12.19–12.20 (non-context, pp. 148) Fig. 12.35 (in context, pp. 154)	Fig. 12.46 See DVD	Fig. 12.54 (non-context, pp. 162) Figs 12.61–12.64 (in context, pp. 165–166) See DVD
Transition time		See DVD	See DVD	Fig. 12.54 (non-context, pp. 162) See DVD
Balance/postural stability		Figs 12.36–12.39 (pp. 155–156)		All procedures in context Figs 12.55–12.64 Also Figs 12.36–12.39

Note Some procedures are difficult to demonstrate in still photography, and are therefore only demonstrated on the DVD. Each procedure challenges several underlying abilities, for example, the hip procedures in standing can be used to challenge trunk balance and coordination. All the challenges should be graded, with an incremental increase in the four movement parameters (force, velocity, length/range and endurance).

Key for figure symbols

	Patient resists and maintains the joint/limb/trunk in the same position.
	Patient moves their limb between two positions.
	Patient moves their limb in one direction.
	Direction of forces applied by the practitioner.
	Direction of forces applied by the practitioner.
	Practitioner resists patient's movement.

Demonstration of challenges: the lower limb

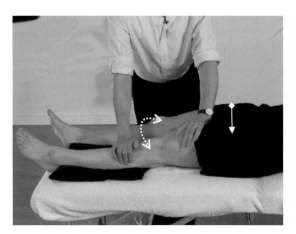

Fig. 12.2 • Co-contraction challenge in rotational plane. Patient stiffens leg and hip and resists internal–external rotation forces imposed by the practitioner.

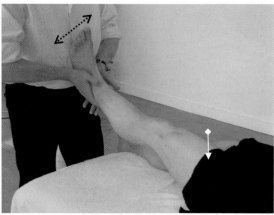

Fig. 12.3 • Co-contraction challenge in lateral plane (adduction-abduction). Patient stiffens leg and hip and resists lateral-medial forces imposed by the practitioner.

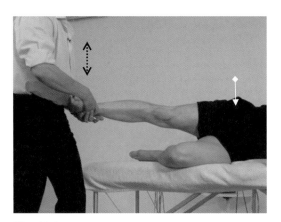

Fig. 12.4 • Co-contraction challenge in the lateral plane. Side lying position, the patient stiffens leg and hip and resists lateral-medial forces imposed by the practitioner.

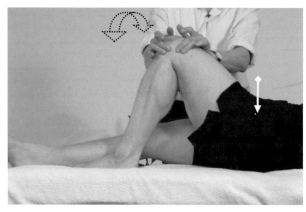

Fig. 12.5 • A variation of co-contraction challenge in lateral plane (adduction-abduction) with hip flexed and foot supported. Patient stiffens leg and hip and resists lateral-medial forces imposed by the practitioner.

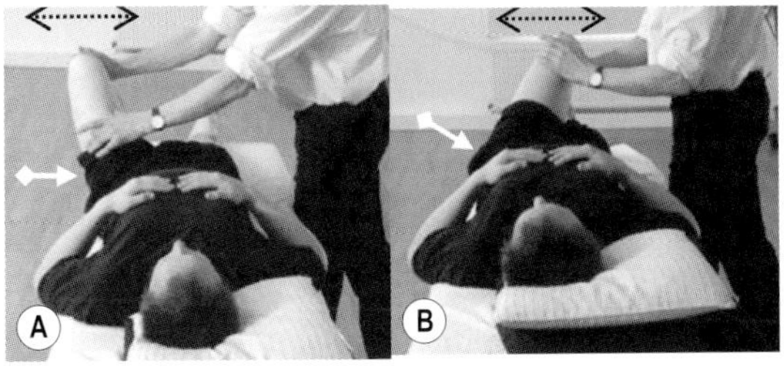

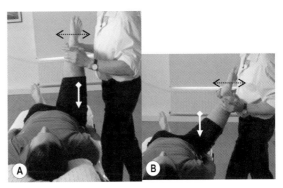

Fig. 12.6 • A variation of co-contraction challenge in lateral plane, adding the length (range) parametric ability. A, In abduction. B, In further adduction.

Fig. 12.7 • Variation of hip co-contraction challenge in the lateral plane. Patient stiffens leg and hip and resists rhythmic meio-lateral forces imposed by the practitioner. A, In neutral position. B, In abduction.

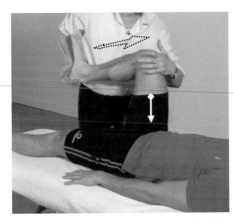

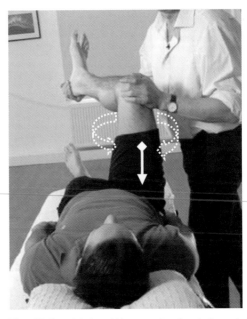

Fig. 12.8 • Challenge of hip co-contraction in the AP plane (flexion–extension). Patient stiffens the leg and hip and resists rhythmic AP forces imposed by the practitioner.

Fig. 12.9 • Variation of hip co-contraction challenge in the rotational plane. The patient stiffens the whole leg and hip and resists the rhythmic rotational forces imposed by the practitioner.

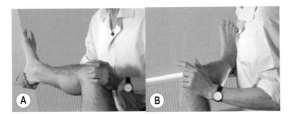

Fig. 12.10 • Varying the length element in rotational co-contraction. Starting point in internal (A) and external (B) rotation.

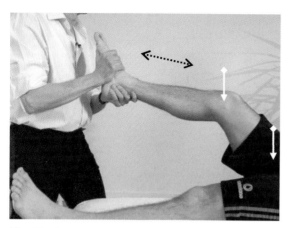

Fig. 12.11 • Co-contraction challenge of the hip and whole leg. The imposed cyclical perturbations can be in single planes (AP, lateral and rotation) or mixed in a random pattern.

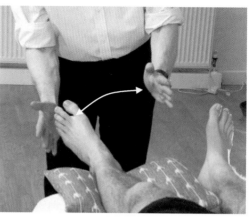

Fig. 12.12 • Reciprocal challenge for the hip in rotational plane. Patient is instructed to oscillate the foot between two positions marked by the practitioner's hands.

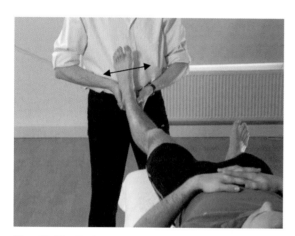

Fig. 12.13 • Reciprocal challenge for the hip in the lateral plane. The patient is instructed to oscillate the foot from side to side while supported by the practitioner. Force challenge can be introduced by practitioner increasing the resistance to the lateral movement.

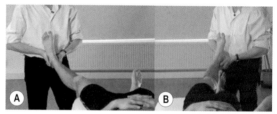

Fig. 12.14 • A length challenge in the lateral plane can be introduced by initiating the movement from different starting positions (**A**, abduction and **B**, adduction). The patient is instructed to oscillate the leg from side to side at the end range.

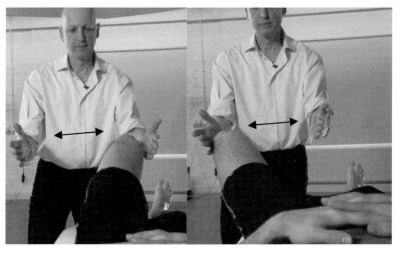

Fig. 12.15 • Reciprocal challenge for the hip in rotation and lateral movement planes. The patient is instructed to oscillate the knee between the two positions marked by the practitioner's hands.

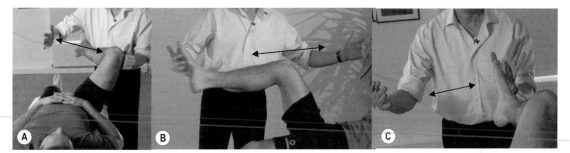

Fig. 12.16 • Variation of reciprocal challenge for the hip. With the foot off the table control of the hip can be challenged in different planes, by instructing the patient to oscillate the knee and the foot between the practitioner's hands. A, lateral, B, AP and C, rotational planes.

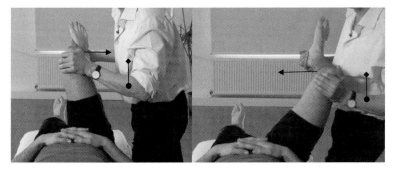

Fig. 12.17 • Reciprocal activation combining force challenge to the hip in the lateral plane. The patient is instructed to cyclically adduct and abduct their leg while the practitioner provides varying levels of resistance.

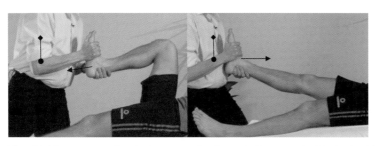

Fig. 12.18 • Reciprocal activation combining force challenge to the hip, in the AP plane. The patient is instructed to rhythmically cycle with their leg against resistance.

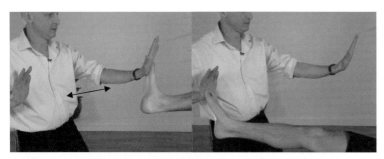

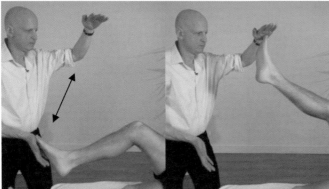

Fig. 12.19 • Reciprocal activation challenge for the leg and hip. Introducing continuous variations in planes of movement and length control. The practitioner starts with simple repetitive patterns and graded, by increasing the velocity of movement, position of, and the distance between the hands. This procedure also challenges single-limb coordination.

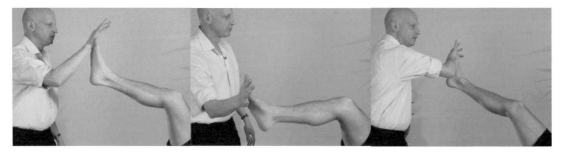

Fig. 12.20 • A coordination challenge for the leg/hip. The patient is instructed to follow the practitioner's hand movement in space. This challenge can be graded by commencing with simple and slow arcs of movement to more complex and faster movement patterns.

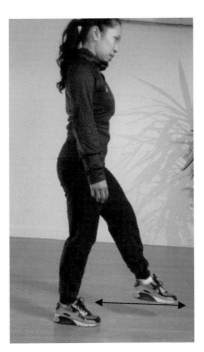

Fig. 12.21 • Swinging the free leg in the AP plane challenges AP co-contraction of the hip on the weight-bearing side.

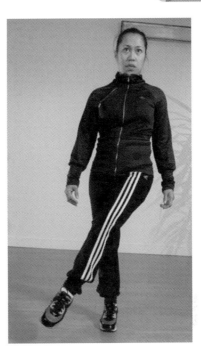

Fig. 12.22 • Swinging the free leg in the lateral plane challenges lateral co-contraction of the hip on the weight-bearing side.

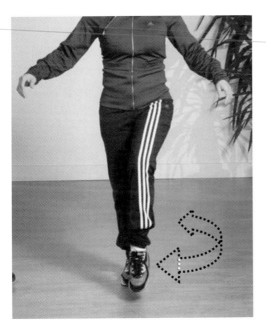

Fig. 12.23 • Swinging the free leg in the rotational plane challenges rotational co-contraction of the hip on the weight-bearing side.

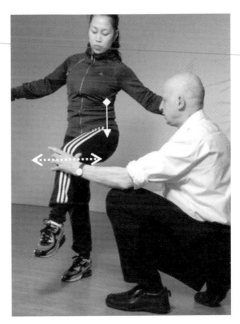

Fig. 12.24 • Co-contraction combined with force challenge to the weight-bearing leg. The patient is instructed to stiffen the free leg and resist the forces applied by the practitioner. The forces can be applied in the rotational and AP plane. The force applied will transfer to the weight-bearing leg.

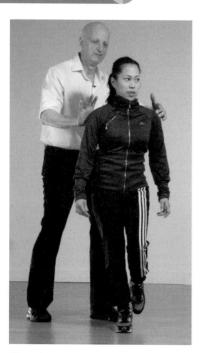

Fig. 12.25 • Co-contraction challenge to the weight-bearing hip and leg. The practitioner applies forces in the AP, lateral and rotational planes either in sequence or randomly.

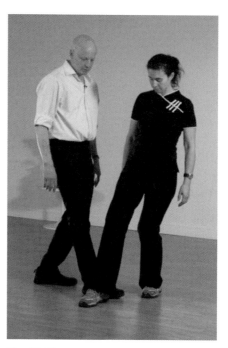

Fig. 12.26 • Reciprocal and length challenge for the hip. The patient is instructed to step over the practitioner's foot. The foot can be placed at different distances to challenge the AP range of movement.

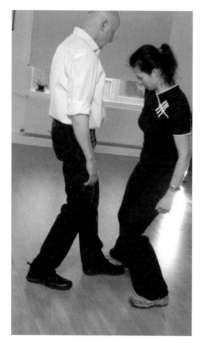

Fig. 12.27 • Reciprocal and length challenge for the hip in the lateral plane (abduction-adduction). The patient is instructed to step over the practitioner's foot. The foot can be placed at different distances to challenge the lateral range of movement.

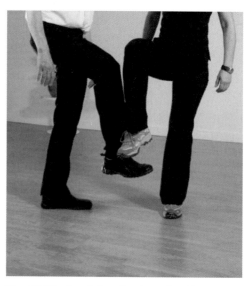

Fig. 12.28 • A variation of reciprocal and length challenge for the hip and leg in the AP plane (can be also performed in the lateral plane). This is achieved by raising the obstacle (foot) over which the patient has to step.

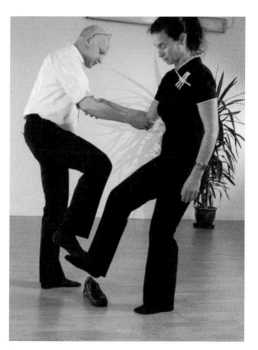

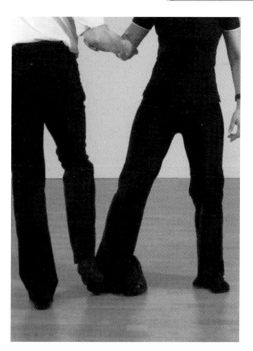

Fig. 12.29 • Reciprocal and force challenge of the hip and leg in the AP plane. The patient steps over an obstacle while the practitioner provides resistance through the foot.

Fig. 12.30 • Reciprocal and force challenge of the hip and leg in the lateral plane. The patient steps over an obstacle while the practitioner provides resistance through the foot.

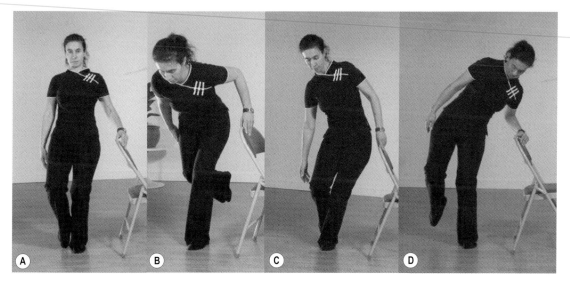

A   B   C   D

Fig. 12.31 • Reciprocal and force challenge for the hip and leg. The patient performs single leg up-down squats. By bending in different directions the forces challenge can be increased on the antagonistic muscle groups. A & B, slight tilting backwards or forwards increases the challenge in the AP plane. C & D, side tilting will increase the challenge in the lateral plane.

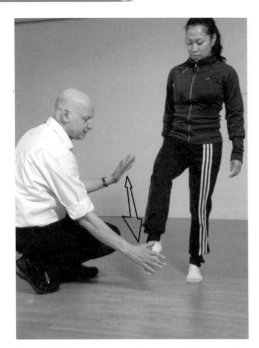

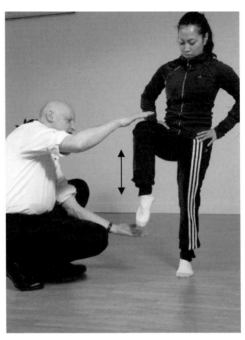

Fig. 12.32 • Reciprocal activation challenge of hip and leg (free leg). The patient moves their foot between the two positions marked by the practitioner's hands. The distance between the hands can be varied to include length challenge.

Fig. 12.33 • Reciprocal activation challenge of hip and leg in the antero-posterior plane (flexion–extension cycles). The patient taps with their foot and knee the practitioner's hands. The distance between the hands can be varied to include length challenge.

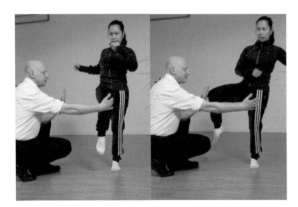

Fig. 12.34 • Reciprocal activation challenge of hip and leg in the rotational plane (flexion–extension cycles). The patient swings their knee between the two positions marked by the practitioner's hands.

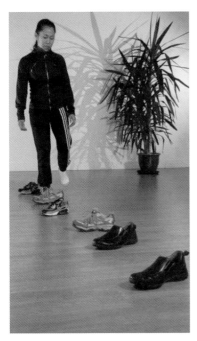

Fig. 12.35 • Multi-limb co-ordination challenge for the legs. Patient walks over obstacles placed randomly on the floor. This can be performed with one leg walking within and the other outside the obstacle course or walking with both legs passing through the obstacle course.

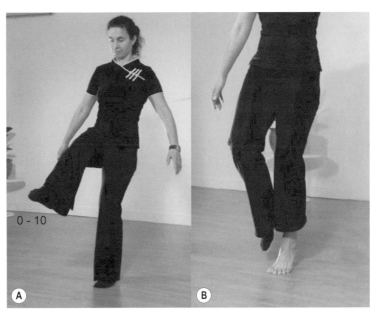

Fig. 12.36 • Balance/postural stability challenge. A, Balancing on the affected side and drawing imaginary numbers from 0-10 with the unaffected side. B, Further challenge to balance can be introduced by standing on the forefoot and drawing the numbers.

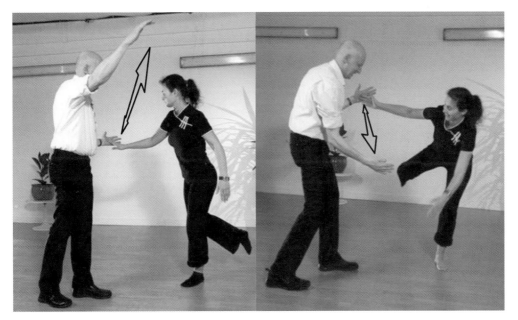

Fig. 12.37 • Balance/postural stability challenge. While standing on one leg the patient moves one hand between two positions marked by the practitioner's hands. A transition time challenge can be added by sudden and rapid changes in the distance between the hands and the planes of movement.

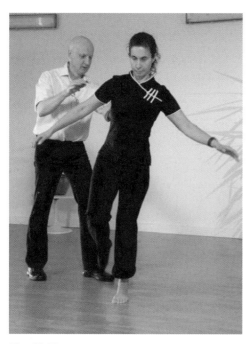

Fig. 12.38 • Unexpected challenge to balance/postural stability can be introduced by multidirectional perturbations provided by the practitioner.

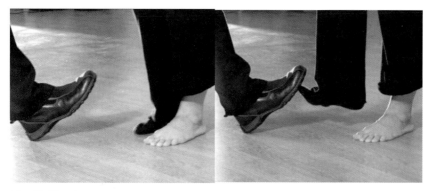

Fig. 12.39 • For more disabled patients balance can be challenged by the patient tapping the practitioner's foot with their un-affected foot. This challenge can be graded by increasing the number of taps the patient has to perform or moving the target further away. This encourages the patient to spend a longer time balancing on the affected side. It can be used to build up the patient's confidence to weight-bear or balance on the affected leg.

Demonstration of challenges: upper limb

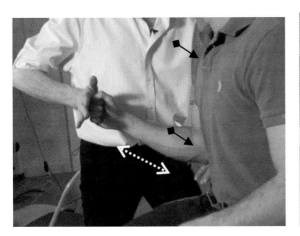

Fig. 12.40 • Co-contraction challenge, shoulder and arm control in the AP plane (flexion–extension of the shoulder). The patient is instructed to stiffen their shoulder/arm and resist the AP movement imposed by the practitioner.

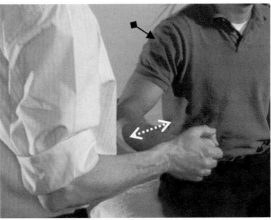

Fig. 12.41 • Co-contraction challenge, shoulder and arm control in the lateral plane (adduction-abduction of the shoulder). The patient is instructed to stiffen their shoulder/arm and resist the lateral plane movement imposed by the practitioner.

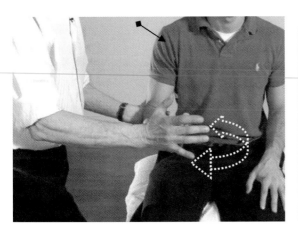

Fig. 12.42 • Co-contraction challenge, shoulder and arm control in the rotational plane (internal–external rotation of the shoulder). The patient is instructed to stiffen their shoulder/arm and resist the imposed rotational forces imposed by the practitioner.

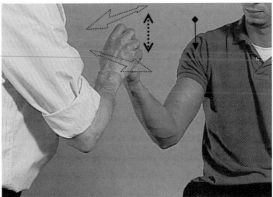

Fig. 12.43 • Co-contraction challenge, shoulder and arm control multidirectional.

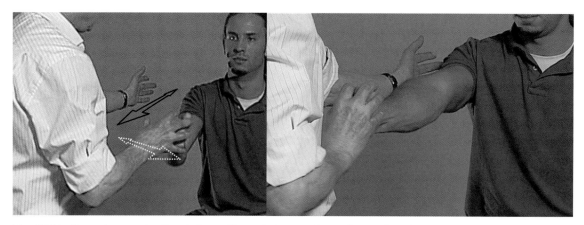

Fig. 12.44 • Dynamic co-contraction challenge. The patient moves the arm in one plane, here in the AP plane. The practitioner introduces perturbations at 90° to that plane. In this challenge the perturbations are in the lateral plane. During the procedure, the practitioner instructs the patient to perform cyclical movement in parallel to the practitioner's outstretched arm.

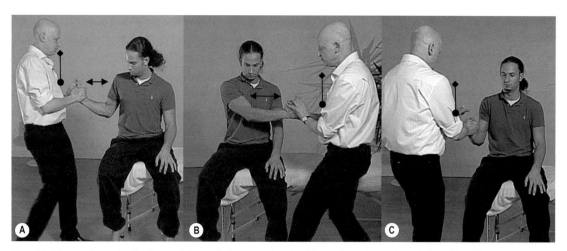

Fig. 12.45 • Reciprocal activation and force challenge to the shoulder and arm in the lateral plane (A & B) and (C) AP planes.

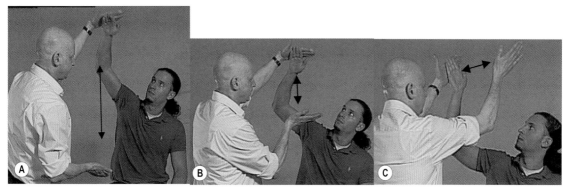

Fig. 12.46 • Reciprocal activation and length challenge, varying length (**A** & **B**) and movement plane (**C**).

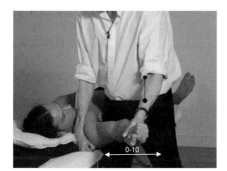

Fig. 12.47 • Functional stretching. The joint is taken to the end-range passively. In this position the patient performs functional movement against the practitioner's resistance. In this example of the shoulder the patient is instructed to perform movements such as waving a flag above head, drawing imaginary numbers from 0-10. The elbow should be locked in extension to ensure the use of the shoulder in the movement.

Demonstration of challenges: the trunk

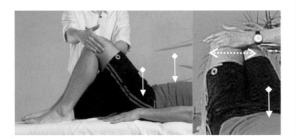

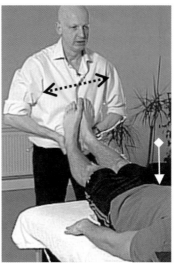

Fig. 12.48 • Co-contraction challenge in rotation control of the trunk. The patient maintains their leg and knee in the position against rotational perturbations applied to the knees.

Fig. 12.49 • Co-contraction challenge of the trunk in the lateral plane. Patient keeps the legs and trunk in line against lateral perturbations applied at the feet.

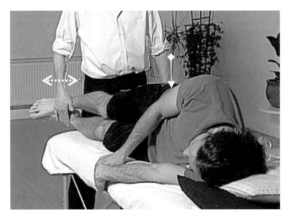

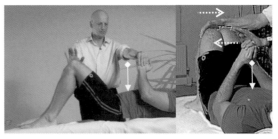

Fig. 12.50 • Co-contraction challenge of the trunk in the AP plane. The patient attempts to keep their trunk and legs in line against AP forces applied at the ankle. This challenge can be performed with the legs straight or with the knees slightly bent which tends to reduce the leverage and forces on the lower back.

Fig. 12.51 • Co-contraction and force challenge of the trunk in the rotational plane. The patient interlocks their fingers and keeps their elbows close to their side. They are instructed to keep the knees and hands in line. The practitioner applies an opposing force on the hands and the knees.

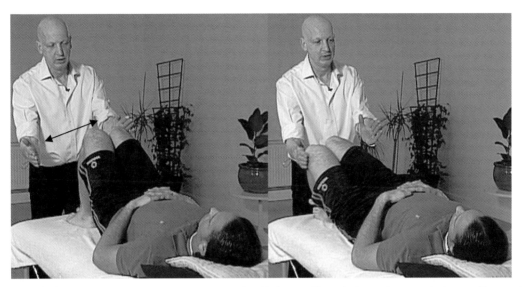

Fig. 12.52 • Reciprocal activation challenge in rotation. Patient oscillates the knees between the two positions marked by the practitioner's hands.

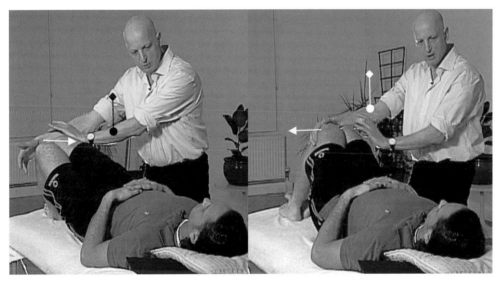

Fig. 12.53 • Reciprocal activation and force challenge in rotational plane. Patient rolls both knees to the sides against the practitioner's resistance. This procedure can be also applied to in the lateral and AP planes, similar to the positions in Figures 12.49 and 12.50.

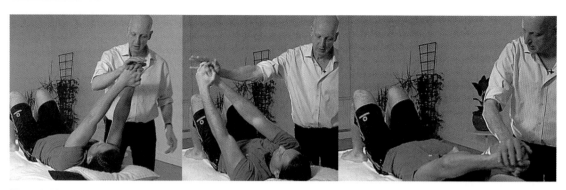

Fig. 12.54 • Transition time challenge between reciprocal activation and co-contraction. The patient follows the practitioner's hands in different movement patterns. During the movement the practitioner suddenly stops the movement and at that point the patient has to co-contract and resist imposed perturbations in different planes. Throughout this challenge the patient should maintain their elbows locked in extension. This ensures that the trunk is recruited during the movement.

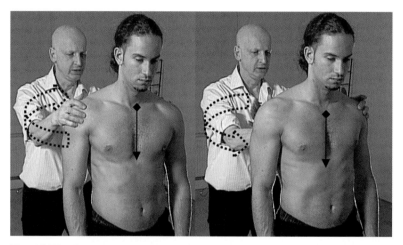

Fig. 12.55 • Co-contraction and force challenge to the trunk in rotation. The patient resists the turning force applied by the practitioner.

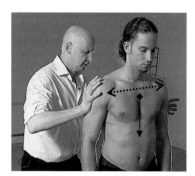

Fig. 12.56 • Co-contraction and force challenge to the trunk in the lateral plane. Same procedure as in Fig. 12.55.

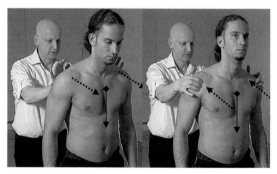

Fig. 12.57 • Co-contraction and force challenge to the trunk in the AP plane. Same procedure as Fig. 12.55. **Note on this procedure:** This procedure can be used to challenge reciprocal activation of the trunk in different movement planes. In this challenge the patient initiates the movement in rotation, lateral or AP planes against resistance provided by the practitioner.

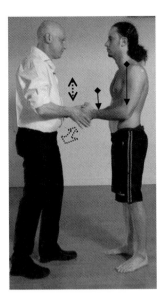

Fig. 12.58 • Co-contraction and force ability challenge in multiple planes. The patient interlocks their fingers and maintains the elbows at right angles and close to their sides. They are instructed to maintain this position, during which the practitioner applies perturbations in different planes. The perturbations can be graded from challenges in one plane, resisting circular movement imposed by the practitioner to more complex and random perturbations in different planes.

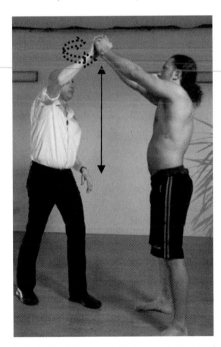

Fig. 12.59 • Dynamic co-contraction control. Patient moves their arms and trunk in the AP plane (flexion–extension), during which the practitioner applies lateral perturbations.

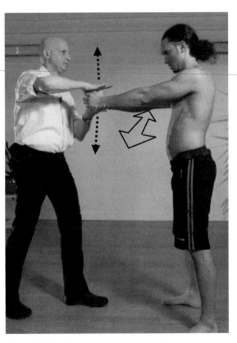

Fig. 12.60 • Dynamic co-contraction in rotation. Patient rotates the hand and trunk in the horizontal plane, during which the practitioner applies perpendicular forces in the AP plane.

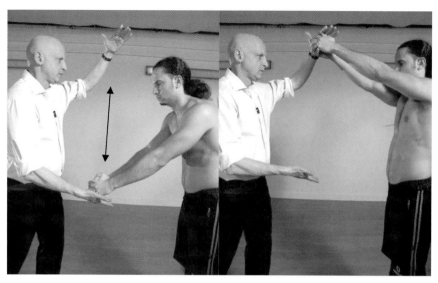

Fig. 12.61 • Reciprocal activation, trunk in AP plane. The patient swings their arms between the two positions marked by the practitioner's hand. It is important that the patient keeps their elbows locked in extension. This will ensure that the trunk is recruited to a greater extent in the movement. When working with patients who suffer from back pain the movement should be in ranges that are pain free. The range can be increased as the patient's condition improves. Often changes in the range can be seen within a few cycles during the session.

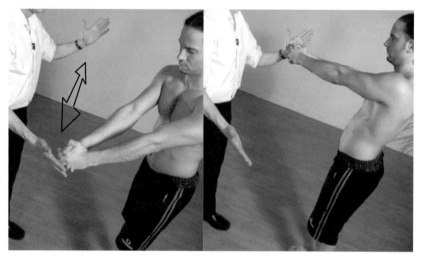

Fig. 12.62 • Reciprocal activation, trunk in lateral plane. Same procedure as in Fig. 12.61. A transition time challenge can be introduced in all this group of procedures by the introduction of sudden changes in the length or plane of movement.

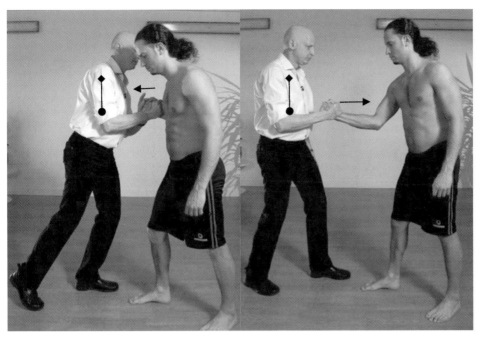

Fig. 12.63 • Reciprocal activation and force control of trunk in the AP plane. The patient pulls and pushes against varying levels of resistance provided by the practitioner.

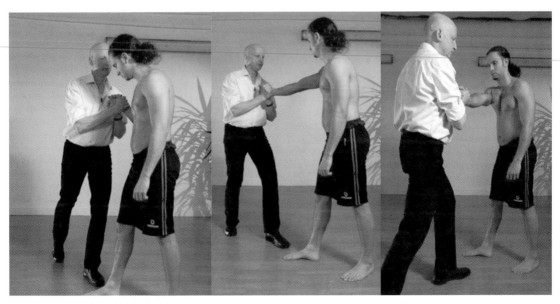

Fig. 12.64 • Reciprocal activation and force control of the trunk in the lateral and rotational planes. Same procedures as in Fig. 12.63. In this group of procedures a transition time element can be added by introducing a sudden change in the resistance force provided by the practitioner.

Optimizing proprioceptive recovery

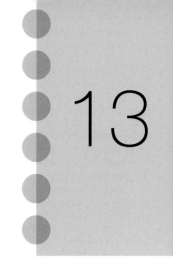

The recovery of proprioceptive ability is a combination of repair and adaptation of the mechanoreceptors and their central representation as well as the repair and adaptation of the tissues in which the receptors are embedded (Ch. 4). These are intrinsic process that are greatly facilitated and optimized by active movement. All of the motor challenges described in Chapter 12 will also stimulate proprioception.

However, some patients may be unable to execute active movement and may, therefore, require passive forms of proprioceptive stimulation. This chapter will explore ways of assessing and facilitating proprioception recovery.

Sensory ability: assessment and challenge

The sensory complexity model discussed in Chapter 4 can be used as a framework for assessing and stimulating proprioception. Three levels of sensory ability were identified:

- Primary proprioceptive ability (position, movement and effort sense)
- Spatial orientation
- Composite sensory ability.

The assessment of composite sensory ability is outside the scope of this book; therefore, the focus will be on proprioception (see Table 13.1 for summary of proprioceptive assessment).

Assessing position and movement sense

All the tests described below should be done with eyes closed (the patient!).

Position sense

This can be assessed by matching the position of the unaffected side to the affected side. For example in the knee, the patient sits with knees flexed at 90 degrees. The practitioner passively moves the *affected* lower leg to a new angle (the subject has to completely relax the leg). The patient has to match this position with the unaffected leg (Fig 13.1). If only the affected leg is available for testing, the practitioner can move the joint to a specific position. The patient has to remember this position and then actively recall it after the practitioner moves the joint to a different position (see DVD, Part 4 sensory assessment).

This assessment bypasses the sense of effort. It might be worth trying the same test but with the patient *actively* moving the affected leg to a particular position and than matching it with the unaffected leg. This would resemble a more real-life situation where proprioception is engaged during active movement (to include the sense of effort).

Movement sense

The therapist moves the affected limb slowly while the patient attempts to mirror the movement with

Table 13.1 Assessment of proprioception

Sensory abilities		
Ability	**Description**	**Assessment**
Static position sense	Ability to perceive the static angle of the joint.	Patient's eyes shut, moves one limb to a particular angle/position. Patient has to move the other limb to match the same position. Test in different angles (Fig. 13.1).
Dynamic movement sense	Ability to perceive the angle of the joint during movement.	Patient's eyes shut, moves one limb. Instruct patient to follow the movement with the other limb (Fig. 13.1). Test in different velocities.
Spatial orientation	Ability to perceive the position of limbs or trunk in space and direction of movement.	Instruct the patient to shut their eyes and move their limb between two targets (Fig. 13.2).

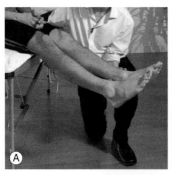
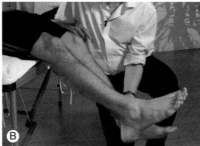
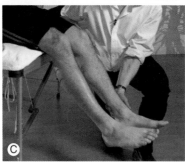

Fig. 13.1 • Assessing position (static) sense. A. starting position, B the leg is moved by the practitioner to a different angle and C the patient matches that position with the opposite leg.

the unaffected limb (same procedure as in Fig. 13.1 but the movement is more continuous, see DVD, Part 4 sensory assessment).

If only the affected limb is available for testing, the therapist can move the patient's limb passively within the movement pairs, e.g. flexion or extension. The patient has to identify in which direction the joint is moving.

Spatial orientation

The patient's eyes are closed.

Assessment

This ability can be assessed by creating two target points: one static and the other moving.

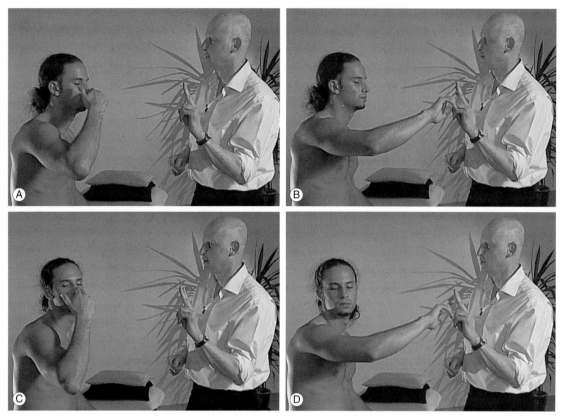

Fig. 13.2 • Assessing spatial orientation. The patient moves their limb between two reference points (A&B). This challenge can be increased by continuously moving the patient's own reference point (head/nose) (C&D).

For example, the dynamic target could be the patient's nose, and the static target point the practitioner's index finger (Fig. 13.2, see DVD, Part 4 sensory assessment). The patient is instructed to touch these two reference points repeatedly with their index finger. The assessment can be made more challenging by instructing the patient to slowly rotate their head during this procedure. Look out for accuracy in reaching the targets and the speed of movement. In this assessment the patient has to build up a spatial map of the position, distances and directions of the limb in relation to the trunk and other limbs.

Another test is to hold the patient's unaffected arm and move it slowly in space in different directions. At the same time the patient has to actively follow and replicate these movements with the affected arm.

Challenging the feedback

The challenging of proprioception is somewhat different to the assessment described above. The challenge can take several forms:
- Any exercise or active movement of the affected limb
- Increasing the afferent stimulation by passive manual approaches
- Reducing the visual feedback.

Any exercise or active movement will stimulate proprioception. This is by far the ideal way to challenge and help proprioceptive recovery. This issue has been discussed at length in Chapters 2 and 4. The next options, passive stimulation and reduced visual feedback, should be used if the patient is unable to execute active movement. Some patients who have a limited ability to execute movement may benefit from the alternate use of passive and active movement.[1]

Manual passive approaches

Generally, passive manual techniques will stimulate proprioception without engaging the efferent and motor elements of the system.

Various groups of proprioceptors will be recruited by different manual techniques.[2] For example, skin mechanoreceptors can be maximally stimulated by dynamic events such as massage and stroking. Maximal stimulation of joint receptors can be achieved by articulation techniques such as cyclical

rhythmical joint movement or oscillation. Proprioceptive stimulation in muscles can be achieved by rhythmic cyclical stretching. Alternatively, the patient can be instructed to contract isometrically while the therapist introduces rhythmic perturbations to the limb. Generally, active–dynamic techniques produce the largest proprioceptive barrage; second to these come passive–dynamic techniques. The influence of the different techniques on proprioception is summarized in Figure 13.3.

Passive manual proprioceptive stimulation may have a role in sensory rehabilitation of severely disabled individuals who are unable to initiate voluntary movement. In healthy individuals, passive stimulation was shown to drive adaptation in the cortical areas involved in preparation and execution

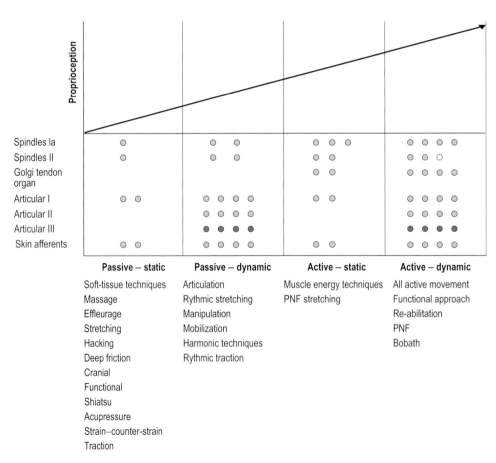

Fig. 13.3 • Summary of the effects of different physical stimulation and the related manual-therapy techniques on proprioception. Shaded circles represent the extent of receptor recruitment.

of movement.[3] A similar finding was demonstrated in patients who had motor hemiplegia with severe motor deficit. This study demonstrated that 4 weeks of proprioceptive training (daily passive motion to the affected wrist), together with standard rehabilitation, promoted further adaptation in sensorimotor centres.[4] However, it is not clear how well this central topographical reorganization translates into improvement in proprioception or motor control.[5]

Proprioception vs. vision

One way of directing attention to proprioception is to instruct the patient to shut their eyes while exercising. It was demonstrated that when subjects learn to balance on a beam, those blindfolded had developed better balance ability than subjects who trained with partial or full vision.[6]

However, when this ability has to be transferred to another movement situation, the source of sensory information during the training is not as important as the similarity between the two tasks (see similarity principle Ch. 5).[7]

Summary points

- Proprioceptive abilities can be assessed by using the sensory complexity model.
- Proprioceptive losses following musculoskeletal injuries can be very small and not detectable by clinical examination.
- Active movement is more effective for stimulation and recovery of proprioceptive losses.
- There are no specific proprioceptive exercises. All exercise will engage the full motor system including proprioception.
- Passive, proprioceptive manual approaches should only be used in the severely disabled individual with severe motor losses.
- Exclusion of vision during movement will drive attention to proprioception.
- The message to the patient with proprioceptive losses: "keep on moving".

References

[1] Lindberg PG, Schmitz C, Engardt M, et al. Use-dependent up- and down regulation of sensorimotor brain circuits in stroke patients. Neurorehabil Neural Repair 2007;21(4):315–326.

[2] Lederman E. The science and practice of manual therapy. Edinburgh: Elsevier; 2005. p. 197–201.

[3] Carel C, Loubinoux I, Boulanouar K, et al. Neural substrate for the effects of passive training on sensorimotor cortical representation: a study with functional magnetic resonance imaging in healthy subjects. J Cereb Blood Flow Metab 2000;20 (3):478–484.

[4] Dechaumont-Palacin S, Marque P, De Boissezon X, et al. Neural correlates of proprioceptive integration in the contralesional hemisphere of very impaired patients shortly after a subcortical stroke: an FMRI study. Neurorehabil Neural Repair 2008;22(2):154–165.

[5] Moore CE, Schady W. Investigation of the functional correlates of reorganization within the human somatosensory cortex. Brain 2000;123(Part 9):1883–1895.

[6] Dickinson J. The training of mobile balancing under a minimal visual cue situation. Ergonomics 1966; 11:169–175.

[7] Mackrous I, Proteau L. Specificity of practice results from differences in movement planning strategies. Exp Brain Res 2007;183(2): 181–193.

Neuromuscular rehabilitation: summary

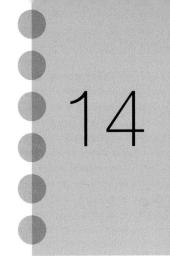

- Neuromuscular rehabilitation aims to help the individual to recover their movement control and optimize their functional capacity.
- It is an inclusive approach that encompasses the cognitive, behavioural and neurophysiological dimensions of the individual.
- The rehabilitation promoted in this book has three basic recurring concepts:
  - It aims to be functional
  - It involves skill/ability-level rehabilitation
  - It uses the learning/adaptation code to optimize motor control changes.

Functional rehabilitation

- *Functional movement* is the movement repertoire of an individual.
- Movement which is out of the individual's experience is termed *extra-functional*.
- Functional rehabilitation utilizes the patient's own movement repertoire to help them to recover their movement losses. It uses actions the patient is already familiar with but can't carry out.
- Extra-functional movement requires a period of learning/training and is, therefore, not ideal for individuals who are in pain or recovering from an injury.

Skill/ability-level rehabilitation

- Neuromuscular rehabilitation can be within a skill and/or ability level.

- Skill is how proficient a person is in performing a particular task.
- Skill depends on practice and a mixture of the sensory-motor and cognitive abilities of the individual.
- Motor abilities are the various control factors that underlie movement.
- At skill-level rehabilitation the patient simply aims to carry out the movements they are currently unable to complete.
- Ability-level rehabilitation (re-abilitation) focuses on specific underlying motor losses which prevent the person from attaining their movement goals.
- Cognition about injury and pain, persistent pain and fear of it, and behavioural factors, are all manageable within skill-level rehabilitation.

The code for neuromuscular adaptation

- Learning, retraining, motor organization to injury and return to functionality depend on the capacity of the motor system to adapt.
- These adaptive processes can be optimized by introducing five principal elements: cognition, activity, feedback, repetition and similarity.
- Cognition involves thinking, rationalizing, memorizing, focusing, being attentive, deciding on actions and understanding the aims and goals of the rehabilitation process.

- Being physically active is important for neuromuscular adaptation. Passive movement approaches are unlikely to be effective in promoting lasting and functional motor control changes.
- Feedback can be intrinsic from proprioception or extrinsic as guidance from the therapist.
- Repetition, repetition, repetition – practice is very important for long-term memory.
- Rehabilitation should use movement patterns that are similar to, and within the context of, the movement being recovered.
- Experiences that possess a higher content of adaptive code elements have a greater potential for promoting long-term changes.

Motor abilities

- Motor abilities can be classified according to their level of motor complexity: parametric, synergetic and composite abilities.
- Parametric abilities are: force, velocity/speed/rate, length, endurance.
- There are two identifiable synergistic control patterns: reciprocal activation and co-contraction.
- Composite abilities are: coordination (fine, single- and multi-limb, and body coordination), balance/postural stability, transition time and motor relaxation.
- Motor ability changes can be observed in musculoskeletal injuries and pain conditions and in patients suffering from central nervous system (CNS) damage.
- There is evidence that motor abilities can be normalized by activities that challenge them specifically.

Sensory ability

- The sensory-motor system is a functional unit.
- Proprioceptive acuity can be affected due to peripheral and/or central causes.
- Musculoskeletal injury can affect the peripheral proprioceptive apparatus while CNS damage will affect the central processing of proprioception.
- Recovery of proprioception comprises both reparative and adaptive processes. As such, it

may have its own inherent recovery period that may take several weeks or months to complete.
- Promoting normal functional movement will help proprioception by facilitating positive sensory-motor reorganization/adaptation. There is no need to specifically target proprioception.
- All exercises are proprioceptive exercises.

The motor system in musculoskeletal injury

- The motor reorganization following injury is a multi-dimensional strategy culminating in postural and movement reorganization aimed at reducing the mechanical stresses imposed on the damaged tissues – in this text it is referred to as *the injury response.*
- The injury response is a positive healthy response and not a motor dysfunction or pathology.
- Acute musculoskeletal injuries should be left alone – the body knows best. The patient should be encouraged to keep active.
- Neuromuscular rehabilitation is useful when the injury response serves no obvious protective function. It includes:
  - Conditions where the injury response has become an adaptive state, such as in chronic recovery from injury or surgery, or conditions where there were movement constraints or immobilization
  - Sensitization conditions where tissue damage has resolved but the patient still experiences pain
  - Injury-related psychological distress that leads to "psychomotor" control losses.
- In the neurological dimension there is no injury specific rehabilitation. A body area is rehabilitated according to its function rather than to the underlying pathology.

Cognition and behaviour

- Cognition, behaviour and movement control are inseparable.
- Helping individuals to modify their injury behaviour and challenging beliefs and attitudes about their condition can facilitate motor recovery.

- Some injuries and pain conditions can be acquired by the way the person uses their body in relation to the physical environment (task behaviour), or by the way in which the person organizes and schedules their physical activities (organizational behaviour, often overuse injuries).
- Guiding individuals in how to modify their task and organizational behaviour could help to prevent musculoskeletal injury and pain.
- Movement control can change solely by cognitive means.

Non-traumatic pain conditions

- Individuals may acquire painful musculoskeletal conditions without traumatic injury.
- Often these conditions develop in low-load, repetitive physical activities (computer use) or in response to psychological distress.
- These conditions often manifest as pain and tender points around the head (tension headache), suboccipital area, neck and neck-scapular muscles (trapezius myalgia) and jaw (bruxism).
- All these conditions share similar processes – inability of the individual to relax, transmission of tension via the neuromuscular system to specific muscles.
- Intervention should be all-inclusive – a combination of cognitive, psychosocial, behavioural, organizational and neuromuscular approaches.
- Focused motor relaxation should be used to train the individual how to relax their painful muscles.
- Transferring the relaxation to functional daily activities is important. Promote relaxation-in-movement.
- The patient's own coping strategies are very important for reducing stress and chronic states of arousal.
- Neuromucular rehabilitation is also about motor relaxation.

Damaged central nervous system

- Many of the principles of neuromuscular rehabilitation can be applied to managing individuals who suffered CNS damage.

- The rehabilitation plan should contain the motor adaptation elements – cognition, activity, feedback, repetition and similarity.
- Keep the training as close as possible to daily functional movement.
- Avoid complex movements that are not within the normal movement repertoire of the individual – train them in something they already know (but can't do).

Further thoughts on motor recovery

- Recovery of motor control is an intrinsic person/nervous-system process.
- This recovery is dependent on psychological, behavioural, neurophysiological and tissue-related factors. Often many of these factors are interrelated.
- The role of neuromuscular rehabilitation is to optimize the recovery of movement control, working with all these factors.
- Rehabilitation is more about facilitating cognitive-sensory-motor processes by providing a stimulating and variations-rich environment. It is not just exercising.
- The movement challenges should be introduced at a level that matches or is above the patient's movement capacity.

Finally

- The only clinical certainty is uncertainty – don't fight it, learn to work with it. You will never know all the answers but you will be expected to provide expert care.
- Complexity rules! Don't become lost in the labyrinth of the neuromuscular system; look at the whole, not at minute details.
- Neuromuscular rehabilitation is a creative process; it is not protocol-based. Every patient is different and presents with new challenges. You will forever have to problem-solve on your feet.
- *Think movement not muscles.*
- There is nothing like one brain to stimulate another.
- Make it fun, interesting and continuously challenging.

Index